Sweet Mysteries of Life

Sweet Mysteries of Life

A Handbook for Naturally Preventing and Healing Diabetes Mellitus

Dr. Akmal Muwwakkil

Copyright © 2010 by Dr. Akmal Muwwakkil.

Library of Congress Control Number: 2009911901
ISBN: Hardcover   978-1-4415-9870-7
        Softcover   978-1-4415-9869-1
        Ebook   978-1-4415-9871-4

All rights reserved. No part of this book may be reproduced or transmitted in any form or by any means, electronic or mechanical, including photocopying, recording, or by any information storage and retrieval system, without permission in writing from the copyright owner.

The author has taken every effort to ensure that the information within this book is accurate and complete to the best of his knowledge. The information within these pages are not to take the place of your physician or other health care provide and is not to diagnose or treat any sickness, illness, disease or health disparity. This publication is strictly for informational purposes and the author nor will the publisher be held liable or responsible for any health conditions, loss, injury, damage or adverse affects from the information or suggestions made in this book.

If the use of any recipes, formulations, or supplements stated in this publication are used the author and publisher are not responsible or liable for any health or allergy needs that may require medical attention. The recipes and formulations are only suggestions and a health care provide should be consulted before the use of any formulations or recipes.

This book was printed in the United States of America.

To order additional copies of this book, contact:
Xlibris Corporation
1-888-795-4274
www.Xlibris.com
Orders@Xlibris.com

CONTENTS

Acknowledgements ... 9
Sweet Mysteries of Life ... 13
Introduction ... 15
Why I Wrote This Book ... 17
History of Diabetes ... 19
Background ... 23
The Making of Diabetes ... 27
Foods and Their Impact on Diabetes ... 33
The Making of Digestion; Absorption, Assimilation, and Elimination Problems in Glucose Control ... 37
    Digestion ... 45
    Gastrointestinal Tract ... 47
    Digestive Processes ... 48
What's Cholesterol Got to Do With It ... 57
Lecithin ... 61
Micronutrient Deficiencies Associated to Diabetes ... 62
Exercise ... 83
Complications of Diabetes ... 85
Overweight/Obesity ... 88
Body Mass Index ... 91
Kidney Disease (Nephrotic Syndrome) ... 94
Neuropathy (Nerve Damage) ... 96
Wound Healing and Foot Ulcers ... 98
Eye Disease Susceptible to Diabetes ... 100
    Cataracts ... 100
    Glaucoma ... 101
    Retinopathy ... 102

Stepping Into the Future With a Healthy Lifestyle Program 103
Enzymes: The Chains of Life 107
The Life of Carbohydrates 111
The Dance of the Maze (Body Mass Index, Glycimic Index, Glycimic Load) 116
Glycemic Load 118
Contribution of Essential Fatty Acids 122
Essential Fatty Acids 126
Alpha-Lipoic Acid 129
Lecithin, The Cell Protector 131
Protein, the Building Blocks of Life 133
    THE EIGHT ESSENTAIL AMINO ACIDS 134
Therapeutic Strategy 141
Protocol of Health Elements for Diabetes 144
Micronutrient 146
    The Power of Vitamin C 151
    The Workings of Vitamin E 152
    Super Foods 154
    Enzyme Therapy 157
    Phytonutrients 161
    Herbal Therapy 161
Acid/Alkaline-Ph balance 165
    Acidic Foods 167
    Alkaline Foods 167
Combining Foods 168
    Fruits 169
    Vegetables 172
    Starches 173
    Fats 173
    Fats/Protein 174
    Protein 174
    Protein/Starches 174
    Sweets 174
Foods to Avoid 176
Healing Foods for Diabetes 179

Diabetic Eating Plan 183
QI Gong 187
A Traditional Chinese Medical look at healing Diabetes 190
QI 194
    Yin/Yang Concept 195
    Organ Network 195
    Nourishing Cycle 196
    Controlling Cycle 196
Traditional Organ Network Chart 198
Traditional Chinese Organ Network 199
    Liver/Gallbladder 199
    Liver 200
    Gallbladder 202
    Heart/Small Intestine 202
    Heart 203
    Small Intestine 203
    Spleen/Stomach/Pancreas 204
    Spleen 205
    Stomach 207
    Lungs 207
    Large Intestine 210
    Kidney 211
    Bladder 216
Case Studies 218
    Study 1 218
    Study 2 219
    QI Gong (Physical Activity) 221
Conclusion 223
References 225

Acknowledgements

I would like to thank the following people for their time, input encouragement and direction in the development of this book.

I would like to first thank God for giving me the strengthen, understanding, power and ability to produce this book in order to assist in the healing of some ones' life.

I would like to thank my parents for their years of my development. As I know they would be proud of this accomplishment and that I am staying the course of my ancestors. With whom I would also like to give honor.

Mrs. Deborah Beasley, was a major contributor in encouraging me to stay the course. As she would say "when is the book coming out."

I would like to thank Ms. Jamie L Smith, who took time out of her scheduler to edit the book.

I would like to acknowledge Mr. Lorenzo Brown the publisher and editor of "Sister 2 Sister" magazine for his challenging comments, ideas, concepts and time he spent editing the book.

Mr. Larry Smith of "Larry Smith's Design" turned my book cover idea and concept into a dynamic visual cover of this book. I will like to thank Mrs. Gayle Miller for assisting in the final editing of this book.

Ms. Lisa Mushaw was an inspiration on many different levels in the development of this book. She was one of the people who aided me in staying on course. I give honor to three of my mentors who guided me over the years, before their passing to understand the work I am here to carry out during my time on earth, which includes Dr. Prem DeBen, Dr. John Chissell and Dr. Phenius P D Vincent Buyck, Sr.

I would especially like to thank all of my clients, and health care professional who provided me the opportunity to be in their presence

and either work with them or on them as part of my life's work on earth.
Thank you all.
May God continue to bless you.

B Well
Akmal Muwwakkil, Ph.D.

"The body has considerable power to heal itself. It is the role of the physician or healer to facilitate and enhance this process, preferably with the aid of natural, nontoxic therapies. Above all, the physician or healer must do no harm."
Michael T. Murray

Sweet Mysteries of Life

A Handbook for Naturally Preventing and Healing Diabetes Mellitus

Sweet Mysteries of Life is a compilation of natural research data that provides information educating consumers on natural methods of reducing and/or eliminating high blood glucose levels. It presents methods of lifestyle changes through conscious eating, exercising, and food supplementation. Sweet Mysteries of Life looks at the relationship between food, environment, emotions and high blood glucose levels, in it ability to aid in the transformation to positive health. Each chapter bring the reader closer to improving their health and longevity by promoting innovative methods of eating, exercising and thinking about their health.

It identifies methods of combining foods for optimum digestion, absorption and assimilation of nutrients to reduce high blood glucose levels, decrease cholesterol, and to improve blood pressure in order to promote health and well being. The key to reversing diabetes is to improve digestion, absorption and assimilation of nutrients.

Sweet Mysteries of Life guide you through understanding of the Glycemic Index to aid in balancing your intake of foods that will slow down the amount of glucose entering your blood at one time. In the supplementation portion of the book you learn the different deficient nutrients that are common amongst diabetics. It shows methods of increasing these nutrients to assist the body in improving its nutritional values resulting in a greater nutritional uptake reducing high blood glucose levels and its complications.

Unlike other books on this subject, Sweet Mysteries of Life takes a step further in providing information from a traditional Chinese prospective. In this section it walks you through the organ network and how they connect to each other. It gives detail about their emotions, structure and relationship to diabetes.

You will find two case studies in the book to show how using the suggested supplements and foods you can reduce and/or eliminate high blood glucose levels.

If you take time and read through the pages of this book you will find that it can assist you in improving your blood sugar levels and over all health.

Introduction

Diabetes has evolved to be today's epidemic level of both type 1 and type 2 diabetes mellitus. Through out the centuries since the Egyptians, diabetes has been classified as genetic inheritance, virus infection, and within the past fifteen years looked at as being related to poor eating habits and lack of exercise. It has also been demonstrated that a lack of breast feeding is also associated with type 1 diabetes. All of these are major contributors to the nutritional deficiencies associated with Diabetes mellitus.

Without breast feeding children are unable to receive the proper antibodies to stabilize their immune systems. This instability leaves them susceptible to infections like the Cox virus, which is linked to type I diabetes. The food industry is no help either; providing poor quality, denatured, overcooked, and processed foods deficient in vital nutrients. These factors contribute to immune deficiencies and obesity which are catalysts for diabetes. Deficiencies in foods are one major reason type 2 diabetes is growing at an epidemic rate. This is the case specifically in the United States and a trend can also so be associated around the world, especially amongst children.

This study will illustrate the relationship between nutritional deficiencies and the development of type I and II diabetes mellitus. It investigates several evidence-based studies that promote the concept and theory of nutritional deficiencies being one of the major causes of diabetes. This research outlines the different nutritional deficiencies and the opportunistic diseases associated with diabetes. Research also identifies the relationship between denatured food, diabetes and obesity that leads to type 2, cardiovascular disease, blindness and other disparities.

As a result of denatured food and the growth of diabetes, this study examines the role of micronutrients, including but not limited to chromium, magnesium, fatty acids, zinc, amino acids and other micronutrients to reduce and/or eliminate high blood glucose levels. It also shows a parable between foods such as sugar, fats, their combinations, and the nutritional effects on the metabolic principles. Research is presented that identifies poor consumption of nutrients that promote either the deficiency of insulin production (type I) or in type 2, insulin resistance.

Why I Wrote This Book

Why it is important to you and your ability to over come diabetes and other contributing disorders.

There are a few books out there discussing the natural methods of addressing diabetes. The difference in my book is that not only do I address the issues but, you will find that I use the words disorder instead of the word dis-ease. The difference is that diabetes is a disorder of the body where the body is suffering from malnutrition due to mal-absorption of nutrients form the foods consumed, which I will discuss later. I will also show you that when you supply the body with the proper nutrients the body will prosper and the disorder will disappear.

Dis-ease on the other hand, is a dis-connection from your spirit and the body is not able to heal. The body heals only because your spirit is what allows us to wake up everyday and perform the activities we do. When the spirit leaves the body there is no more life force and the cells no longer are able to perform their task and the oxygen is not able to replenish the lungs. The last thing a person does before going into the next world is to breathe their last breath out with the sound of "Ha". When that happens the life force is gone.

I wrote this book because I watched my parent and relatives take medication all their lives and some of them had such tremendous side effect from the drugs they took. My mother who was a healer would take herbs until she was not able to see (glaucoma) and had to rely on pharmaceutical medicine. I remember visiting her in the hospital days before her spirit guide came to take her home. She told my father, sister and myself that they were killing her and we needed to take her out of the hospital. Well three day later she passed to the other side. The same thing happened to my father who went into the hospital for an in and out mild procedure. I also said they were killing him. A few days after I visited pop (my father) he passed in the hospital from sepsis (waste poisoning of the blood). One thing my mother told me was to continue her and my grandmother's IRA from my mother, who it was pass down from generations to generations of women in my family, work of healing people. My journey began when I was 9 years old and got serious during my twenties and in my thirties I began to assist family, friends, and the community with the knowledge I learned from Dr. Yang (Traditional Chinese Medicine 1970's), Master Heg Robinson (Tai Chi, Herbal medicine), Saul Davis (International School of Shiatsu, Japanese medicine), Dr. Yen Xain (Tui Na—Traditional Chinese Bodywork) also the Traditional Academy of Chinese Medicine in Bejing China, my mentor, friend and father figure Dr. Pathenis Byck who introduced me to the world of viralology, homeopathics and herbal research and Dr. Prime De Ben who walked me through the understanding of how to address HIV/AIDs with nutrition and herbal therapy.

Because of these teachers who were and are masters in their field and have shared their knowledge and wisdom with me over the years, has provided me with the ability to research the information and provide you with an alternative to western medicine. I am not saying that if you need western medicine not to use it, I am saying don't be afraid to make a change and watch the change as it happens. If you find a complementary alterative health care worker that has the understanding and background in the tradition of healing then try them and see what happens. The interesting thing is that herbal, homeopathic, spiritual medicine and manipulation therapies were around centenary before allopathic medicine. According to Barbara Starfield, M.D. in an article published in the Journal of the American Medical Association (JAMA), she states, "that physician error, medication error and adverse events from drugs or surgery kill 225,400 people per year." Of that number 106,000 are related to adverse drug affects. [1]

History of Diabetes

"It is much more important to know what sort of patient has the disease than to know what sort of disease the patient has!"

Dr. William Osler (1849-1919)

Diabetes Mellitus is no stranger to us dating back as far as the ancient Egyptians in 1550 BC, where Hesi Ra used natural healing arts formulas of beer (fermented hops), water from the bird pond, cucumber flowers, animal, minerals, and vegetables as part of treatment to manage the disease.[2,3] Later in 500-600 BCE the father of Ayurvedic (medicine of India) medicine Susruta, described diabetes as a disease and distinguishing the difference between the types of diabetes is credited to Charaka a famous Ayurvedic practitioner. His information identified the differences by age groups, which is now promoted as type 1 or type 2 diabetes.[4]

The Greek physician Aretaeus of Cappadoccia described diabetes as "the melting down of flesh and limbs into urine"[5] Aretaeus named the illness "Diabetes" meaning "siphon or run", referring to chronic polyuria. In the first century A.D. Galen of Pergamum, a Greek physician diagnosed diabetes as a kidney disease, which today is well related to modern research. According to "The Treatment of Diabetes Mellitus with Chinese Medicine", around BCE, Paul of Aegina, described dypsacus (a term referring to the tremendous thirst experienced by those with diabetes) as a weakness of the kidneys combined with excessive dampness produced by the body. His recommendation for the disease was to consume a decoction of potherbs, endives, lettuce, rock/fish, the juice of knotgrass, and elecampane in dark wine with dates and myrtle. [6]

In 1776, Matthew Dobson established the first test to measure the amount of sugar in the urine, where he correlated the metabolism of carbohydrates with the disease and sugar in the urine. During 1869 Paul Langerhans a German medical student in his dissertation discussed the two systems of cells where only one of them secreted pancreatic enzymes, which was later known as the Islets of Langerhans. Late in 1889, Oskar Minkowski and Joseph von Mering at the University of Strasbourg, France, removed a dog's pancreas to show the relationship between the rise in glucose levels and the glucose and ketones found in the urine resembling diabetes. The 1900's brought about major results in the ability to cure diabetes with the first injectable glycosuia extract developed by Georg Zuelzer of Germany in 1908; however the injection caused too many side effects. Other potential diabetes cures came along in 1910, including the "Diabetes Fad diet" comprised of the Oat-cure (as we will see later oats are a major source of chromium), the milk diet, the rice cure, potatoes therapy and even opium used in the United States until 1910. [7,8]

During the years from 1910 to 1920 two leading diabetes specialist emerged on the scene. Fredrick Madison Allen and Elliot P Joslin believed "diabetes to be the best of the chronic disease's because it was clean, seldom unsightly, not contagious, often painless and susceptible to treatment. However, three years after studying diabetes in 1913 Allen published "Studies Concerning Glycosuria and Diabetes" a book that revolutionized the treatment for diabetes. Later in 1919 he, published another work on diabetes, "Total Dietary Regulation in the treatment of Diabetes", citing exhaustive case records of 76 of the 100 diabetes patients he observed. Glycosuria's research, lead him to become the director of diabetes research at the Rockefeller Institute. He also established the first clinic in the United States located in New Jersey to treat diabetes, hypertension, and Bright's disease. The wealthy and desperate patients flocked to him.

An interesting turn of events occurred on October 31, 1920 when Dr. Frederick Banting conceived the idea of researching the relationship between insulin and diabetes after reading Moses Barron's "The Relation of the Islets of Langerhans to Diabetes with Special reference to Cases of Pancreatic Lithia sis" in the November issue of Surgery, Gynecology and Obstetrics. Over the next year Dr. Banting teamed with Charles Best, James Collip, and J.J.R. Macleod and continued to research using a variety of different extracts on de-pancreatized dogs. A break through came in 1921 when Banting and Best discovered that by extracting substances from the dogs pancreas and using these substances on de-pancreatized dogs that the substance would lower the dog's blood glucose levels. They went on to begin extracting insulin from bovines and using it with success. During that year Banting presented his paper "The Beneficial Influences of Certain Pancreatic Extracts on Pancreatic Diabetes' to the American Physiological Society at Yale University. The conclusive research on this protein known today as insulin was first administered to Leonard Thompson a fourteen year old boy on January 11, 1922 of Toronto Canada. By February the treatment was claimed to be a success. Another significant turn of events occurred in 1922 when Eli Lilly and Company and the University of Toronto were contracted to mass produce insulin in North America. Dr. Banting and colleague Professor Macleod were awarded the Noble Prize in Physiology of Medicine. The award was shared between Banting, Maclaeod, and Collip.

In 1930, protamine zinc insulin was introduced. However, during the 1940's a link was made between diabetes and long-term complications as nephropathy (kidney) and retinopathy (eye). The break through discovery in 1944 of the standard insulin syringe assisted in making diabetes management more uniform. In 1949, the first diabetes association was born in Canada by Dr Best known then as Diabetic Association of Ontario. Later it became known as the Canadian Diabetes Association and in 1953 the association was firmly established. Banting founded the first camp for children with diabetes during that same year in Canada. The 1950's introduced the lente series insulin, and in 1955 oral drugs where introduced to assist in lowering blood glucose levels. During 1955 Dr. Frederick Sanger who later in 1958 was awarded the Nobel Prize in Medicine discovered the complete amino acid sequence of polypeptides linked to diabetes.

The 1960's brought about major developments in the quest to understand and treat diabetes. The first home glucose testing kit was developed to identify levels of sugar in urine, which improved glycemic control. The University of Manitoba in Canada preformed the first successful human pancreas transplant leading the way for more then 11,000 pancreas transplants world wide with over 1,000 new transplants each year. [9] 1969 brought about the discovery of proinsulin by Donald

F. Steiner, who showed that insulin is actually synthesized as a larger precursor molecule.[10]

As medical sciences moved into the 70's an insulin meter and insulin pump were developed. Also laser surgery was introduced to treat, assist in slowing down and/or preventing blindness in some diabetics. During the span of time from the 1960's through the 1970's the advancement in chromatography improved the purity of insulin. Introduction of biosynthetic insulin in 1983 was the first recombinant DNA technology insulin made from this process. With this process increasing the purity of insulin and the decrease in the size of injection needles has made subcutaneous insulin injections more comfortable.

Background

"The deviation of man from the state in which he was originally placed by nature seems to have proved to him a prolific source of disease."

> Edward Jenner an inquiry into the causes and
> Effects of the Variolae Vaccinae or Cow Pox (1798)

Diabetes is the sixth leading cause of death in the United States, taking the lives of 224,092 people in 2002[11]. Diabetes mellitus is a multi-digestive disorder associated with nutritional deficiencies, viral infections, and family genetics affecting 23 million people in the United States, including 14.6 million diagnosed, with another 6.2 million people undiagnosed 20 and older.[12] It affects 186,000 children, adolescents and people under the age of 20 in the United States[13], accounting for about one in 400 to 600 children and adolescents with type 1 diabetes, representing 0.22% of the people in this age group.[14]

According to the World Health Organization (WHO) 220 million people worldwide have diabetes. WHO has estimated the growing epidemic of diabetes will double by 2030, with major concerns in developing countries, including population growth in aging, obesity, unhealthy eating habits and sedentary lifestyles.

Another concern is the impact the increasing epidemic of childhood type 2 diabetes has on the future generations. There will be a 42% increase in diabetes, from 51 to 72 million, in the developed countries and a 170% increase, from 84 to 228 million, in the developing countries. Thus, by the year 2025, 75% of people with diabetes will reside in developing countries, as compared with 62% in 1995. The countries with the largest number of people with diabetes are, and will be in the year 2025, India, China, and the U.S. There are more women than men with diabetes, especially in developed countries. In the future, diabetes will be increasingly concentrated in urban areas." [15]

Diabetes is a multi-biochemical deficiency disease causing major digestive health disorders. The body's ability to manage and balance sugar metabolism by the cells is reduced, causing high blood glucose levels. As a result disruption and damage of the pancreas's beta cells and liver's alpha cells in type 1 diabetes; where the pancreas is unable to manufacture insulin and type 2 where the cells become resistant to insulin. Insulin is a hormone produced by the pancreas. It converts sugars and starches into glucose and other elements such as proteins, lipids, minerals, vitamins and amino acids into usable nutrients the cells can use. The cells are then able to digest, absorb, and assimilate for daily nourishment. Insulin is comprised of 51 Amino acids including 30% Leucine, 21% Glutamic acid, Glycine, Glutathione, 12% Tyrosine, Cysteine, Methionine, 8% Histidine, 3% Arginine, 2% Lysine, Phenylalanine, Proline, Peptide, and B3 Niacin.[16]

Type 1 diabetes is referred to as Insulin Dependent Diabetes Mellitus (IDDM). This form of diabetes usually occurs before the 30th birthday and has been referred to as juvenile onset diabetes. IDDM is an autoimmune deficiency disease where the immune system attacks and destroys the pancreas's insulin producing alpha and beta cells. Viruses like the Enteroviruses (coxsackieviruses, polioviruses, and echoviruses), environmental factors, poor eating habits, possibly genetic factors and a lack of breastfeeding are also major links to type 1 diabetes. Type 1 diabetes can slowly mature for several years before affecting a person over 30. With IDDM a person has to take daily insulin injections to maintain a healthy blood glucose level.

Juvenile onset diabetes is normally Insulin Dependent Diabetes Mellitus, which affects 176,500 young people under the age of 20, making them 0.22 % of the population. This averages, out to be 1 in every 400 to 600 children and adolescent developing diabetes during their youth.[17] However, recent reports indicate that 8-45 % of children with newly diagnosed diabetes have type 2 diabetes[18]. This means that Juvenal diabetes is changing to insulin resistance and growing rapidly within our future generation.

When the cells of the body are unable to absorb glucose it results in high blood glucose level, which renders either type 1 or type 2 diabetes mellitus. Between 90 and 95% of the people over the age of 20 with diabetes mellitus have type 2, making it 8% of the population, and an additional 800,000 new cases diagnosed each year. It develops in the population of people over the age of 40 and is common amongst persons 55 and older. Type 2 diabetes is more prevalent within the African American, Hispanic American, Native American Indian, Asian and Pacific Island Americans communities than the European American population. Non-Hispanic Whites account for 13.1 million or 8.7% of the population over the age of 20 diagnosed with diabetes. Non-Hispanic Blacks account for 3.2 million or 13.3% of the population over 20 diagnosed with diabetes.

Among Hispanic/Latino Americans, Mexican Americans are 1.7 times more likely to have diabetes. This factor, in comparison to all Hispanic/Latino American groups makes them about 2.5 million or 9.5% of the population age 20 and older with diabetes.[19] American Indians and Alaska natives account for 99.500 or 12.8% of the population with diabetes of the age group 20 and above. American Indians and Alaska natives are 2.2 times more likely to have diabetes then no-Hispanic whites.

The majority of people with Type 2 diabetes are either overweight or obese. Studies indicate that approximately 80 to 90% of type 2 diabetics are obese.[20] Type 2 diabetes is insulin resistant, where the cells lose their ability to respond to the insulin signals. This significantly elevates blood glucose levels causing several different complications. Excessive glucose in the blood stream causes a domino effect resulting in complications such as eye, kidney and cardiovascular diseases, amputation of the lower limbs, edema, nerve damage, cancer, infections of many types, and un-healing leg ulcers. Statistics are showing one-third of the new Type 2 diabetes cases are children and adolescents who are overweight or obese. Research identifies the change of hormones during puberty as a period causing insulin resistance, which is an important factor in the development of type 2 diabetes in children.[21] Type 2 diabetes mellitus has been recorded in children as young as 4 years old.[22] Dietary factors that contribute to type 2 diabetes include ingesting excessive amounts of processed, overcooked, fast, and denatured foods. Additionally lack of physical activity cause an increase in fat cells (adipose tissue) as they accumulate around their abdomen.

Whether it be type 1 or type 2 diabetes, cells are not able to extract glucose from the blood or unable to absorb nutrients from foods in order to maintain a healthy metabolic balance. This results in mal-absorption leading to malnutrition. Malnutrition creates other health disparities including but not limited to cardiovascular, obesity, and renal failure.

The Making of Diabetes

"When love is on the field, fear must retreat. The whole thing about Soul is survival. Taking care of our health is one of the strongest aspects of survival here."

Harold Klemp

Medical science in the past has only considered the cause of diabetes as genetic. However, modern research now indicates that genetics are not the major cause of diabetes. Environmental factors and dietary habits have proven to promote a greater risk for developing type 1 diabetes than genetics. Julian Whitaker, MD confirms genetic factors are not the primary cause of type 1 diabetes, in her book "Reversing Diabetes". She discusses a set of twins in relationship to diabetes. Dr. Whitaker demonstrates that one twin can develops diabetes, where the other twin is not susceptible to contracting diabetes. She stated, "Only 25 to 50% and not 100% of the time does the other twin develop diabetes. In fact, 85% of all patients with type 1 diabetes have no family history of diabetes. This indicates that diabetes is not inherited however family history can increase a person's risk of developing it." [23]

Michael Murray ND backs up this claim by stating, "We find it interesting that in most medical texts, diabetes organizations and doctors tend to consider type 1 diabetes primarily a genetic disorder. We want to be very clear that while genetics factors may predispose the insulin-producing cells to damage through either impaired defense mechanisms, immune system sensitivity, or some deficiency in tissue regeneration capacity, genetic factors alone account for only a very small percentage of people who develop type 1 diabetes-perhaps as little as 5 to 10 percent of all cases." He continues by stating, "dietary and other environmental factors are the chief factors that ultimately will determine whether the disease will develop." [24]

The environmental impact of viruses on children is a consistent source of type 1 diabetes causing the immune system to attack its beta cells. A number of studies have shown type 1 diabetes being linked to viral infections like Enteroviruses.[25] The Enteroviruses and rotaviruses[i] develop in the gastrointestinal system, due to a lack of healthy micro flora in the intestinal tract, which is a major part of the immune system. "All of these viruses replicate in the gut and stimulate the gut immune system, which may activate the insulin-specific immune cells to seek out and destroy beta cells. These viruses and others can also infect pancreatic beta cells, causing the white blood cells to attack and destroy the beta cells in an attempt to kill the virus", stated Michael Murray, ND. [26]

When intestinal micro flora is deficient, the body is unable to maintain a healthy gut immune system environment where nutrients from foods are absorbed and assimilated into the blood stream. The impairment of the small intestine flora increases the risk of not only type 1 diabetes, but also yeast (Candida albicans also known as thrush). Many infants suffer with recurrent ear infections and constipation when introduced to cow's milk formulas. Such foods containing gluten may also cause celiac disease,[27] It can set the stage for viruses including but not limited to chicken pox, measles, polioviruses, etc. Research has established that children who are exposed to cow's milk at a young age are 1.5 times at risk to type 1 diabetes, ear infections, diarrhea and constipation.[28,29,30] In Georgetown Universities research, cow's milk was found to be responsible for 30% of children's ear infections. They noticed when the children stopped drinking cow's milk formula 86% of the ear infections improved.[31]

The study, at the University of Helsinki in Finland, illustrates the effects of cow's milk verses mother breast milk antibodies in type 1 diabetes. "The study involved 697 newly diagnosed diabetic children, 415 sibling-control children, and 86 birth-date- and sex-matched

---

[i] Enterovirus is a virus that enters the body through the gastrointestinal tract and thrives there, often moving on to attack the nervous system. The Enterovirus includes polioviruses, coxsackie viruses, and echoviruses;MedicineNet.com; www.medterms.com

population-based controls. The research reported that high IgA antibodies levels to cow's milk formula were associated with a greater risk of type I diabetes in infants on a cow's milk based formula as reported during the 59th Annual American Diabetes Association conference. The study showed mothers' breast milk provided the needed nutritional values to promote a healthy gut immune system, warding off diabetes and other disparities; where cow's milk promotes type 1 diabetes by reducing nutrients and antibodies needed to develop healthy immunity.[32] "Unfortunately, due too many factors only 29% of all mothers and 19% of black mothers in the United States breastfeed until the recommended age of 6 months." stated Michael Murray, ND. He goes on to say, "Breast-feeding not only can help prevent the development of food allergies, and it also is vitally important in protecting against Enteroviruses and rotavirus infections and promotes the proper gut micro flora".[33] He also comments that infants exposed to cow's milk are not the only ones at risk of type 1 diabetes, but the ingestion of cow's milk by a person of any age is susceptible to developing type 1 diabetes.[34]

Linking cow's milk to diabetes suggest an autoimmune deficiency disorder, which implies that cow's milk disrupts the pancreas's ability to manufacture and maintain the balance of the beta cells, rendering a child susceptible to type I Insulin Depend Diabetes (IDDM). IDDM is when an individual requires insulin to avoid life-threatening ketoacidosis,[ii],[iii] which would cause a massive autoimmune attack on the B-cells of the pancreas. A condition known as insulitis occurs and active T-lymphocytes infiltrate the islet of Langerhans resulting in the destruction of the pancreas.

On the other hand, type 2 diabetes centers around the consumption of food. Overweight, obese people live sedentary lifestyle, which is demonstrated in the study of the Pima Indian migration. In his research, Peter H. Bennett, MD compared the changing lifestyles of the Pima Indians who migrated to Arizona and consumed a western diet with the Pima Indians living in Mexico who consumed traditional foods containing fresh fruits and vegetable, used wild medical plants,

---

[ii] A compound that is both a ketone and acid. Ketone
[iii] Kentone any of the three compounds acetoacetic acid, acetone, and the beta derivative of hyroxybutyric acid which are normal intermediates in lipid metabolism and accumulate in blood and urine in abnormal amounts in conditions of impaired metabolism (diabetes mellitus).

preformed daily physical labor and lived without modern household conveniences. In the study Bennett exhibited how 70% of the Arizona Pima Indians living in the United States were obese, with a 22% rate of type 2 diabetes, compared to the Mexico Pima Indians who rarely had a case of diabetes and only had a 10% obesity rate.[35] When the Pima Indians of Arizona returned to a traditional eating habit along with performing physical activity their blood sugar levels and weight reduced dramatically. The research evidence demonstrates food consumption and physical activity are the primary factors in type 2 diabetes. Organizations such as the National Institute of Health (NIH) have recognized the fact that genetics have less of an effect on type II diabetes than diet and physical activity to the point where they are educating the Pima Indian children about healthy lifestyles and physical activity. However, not only has NIH looked at diabetes in that manner, other organization over the past years such as the American Diabetes Association have been promoting healthy lifestyles to reduce the epidemic of obesity and type II diabetes.

Another research study conducted by Frank B. Hu, MD, of Harvard School of Public Health, Boston Massachusetts appeared February 2002 in the Annuals of Internal Medicine linking a western typical diet to the development of diabetes. In the study 42,000 men ages 40 to 75 where divided in 2 groups and tracked over a period of 12 years. One group consumed fruits, vegetables, whole grains, fish and poultry, and the other group consumed red meat, processed meat, high-fat dairy products, refined grains and sweets. At the conclusion of the study researchers found 16% (1,321) men, who consumed an unhealthy, poor quality diet to develop type 2 diabetes. The research demonstrated how food consumption changed the physiological conditions of the two groups of men, where the men who consumed the poor diet had a higher risk of contracting type 2 diabetes then the men who maintained a natural eating habit.[36]

As it is shown in these studies, type 2 diabetes is directly related to the quality and quantity of food consumed. Much of type 2 diabetes is related to the understanding of food consumption. Even when we look at genes, it still boils down to the heritage of genes, "food genes", and the eating habits that have been passed down from one generation to another. In some cases families with histories of diabetes, were on public assistance or fixed incomes, had large families or low wage jobs and all too often, were faced with having to buy and eat what they could. Under such circumstances, they had no knowledge of food and its values and would consume advertised products. The ancestors of many diabetic were farmers who cultivated and cooked their food, however, as they migrated and the inner cities grow, so did the food manufactures and processed foods increased and more of these people began to eat processed foods, passing this tradition down from generation to generation. Now the majority of the food is processed and a lot less home cooked meals are being prepared. With this increase of processed and fast foods our society have loss its cooking skills resulting in overweight, obesity and diabetes.

The quality of the food consumed today is worse then 200 or 300 hundred years ago. The minerals in the earth are depleted reducing foods nutritional values, inhibiting their absorption, interfering with the small intestine micro flora, creating abdominal distention, leaky gut syndrome, adiposity, overweight, and obesity resulting in diabetes. The harmful chemicals used reduce the ability to maintain the integrity of the organ system and the immune system. Also the foods we consume are overcooked lacking in enzymes. We also improperly gulp food rather chew it. We also diluted our food by drinking while eating, eat under emotional stress, and have poor food combining habits. These practices decrease the ability of the body to metabolize foods and maintain health causing nutritional deficiencies resulting in overweight conditions, obesity and eventually develop into type 2 diabetes.

The impairment of metabolism increases the adipose tissue, a specialized white or brown connective tissue functioning as a primary fat (triglycerides) storage site promoting obesity, a major risk factor of type 2 diabetes. Much of the relationship between obesity and diabetes is the consumption of food, digestion, absorption, assimilation, elimination and lack of exercise. Obesity results from deficiency of adiponectin[iv] a hormone secreted by the adipose tissue to improve insulin's sensitivity to lower triglycerides.[37] In the journal Diabetes, published by the American

---

[iv] Adiponectin (also referred to as Acrp30, apM1) is a protein hormone that modulates a number of metabolic processes, including glucose regulation and fatty acid catabolism. Adiponectin is exclusively secreted from adipose tissue into the bloodstream and is very abundant in plasma relative to many hormones. Levels of the hormone are inversely correlated with body mass index (BMI). The hormone plays a role in metabolic disorders such as type 2 diabetes, obesity and atherosclerosis.

Diabetes Association, it reported a study on how the Pima Indians high plasma levels of adiponectin where associated with the reduction of type 2 diabetes as it increased insulin sensitivity.[38]

There has been a dramatic increase in overweight conditions and obesity in the past 20 years in the United State, which accounts for 65% of the adult population being overweight and 31% of them categorized as obese. According to the National Health and Nutrition Examination Survey (NHANES) our youth population is not far behind adults as we witness increasing numbers of children who are overweight and obese. The survey shows there has been a steady growth in childhood obesity between the years of 1976 through 2004 where obesity increased from 5.0% to 13.9% in children ages 2-5; youth 6-11 obesity rates grow from 6.5% to 18.8% and in the 12-19 year old group the increase was from 5.0% to 17.4%. The prevalence of childhood obesity increases the risk of children growing into adults being obese and contracting type 2 diabetes. [39]

Foods and Their Impact on Diabetes

"Our advice about the health benefits of diet based largely on food plants-fruits, vegetables, and grains-has not changed in more than 50 years and is consistently supported by ongoing research. On the other hand, people seem increasing confused about what they are supposed to eat to stay healthy."

Marion Nestle Food Politics

According to the United States Department of Agriculture (USDA), in 1996 the average American spent 40% of their food budget on fast and junk foods away from home. They entitled this report "Away from Home Food"; the report documents the relationship between consumers and their consumption of foods in restaurants and other eating establishments. As the population grew so did their willingness to eat out more regularly. The Away From Home Food report tracked the population's eating out habits starting in 1970 where the population spent 25% of their household budget on fast foods until 1996 where it increased by 15%. [40] Cahterine E. Woteki, Acting under Secretary for Research, Education and Economics stated "Seventeen years ago, by comparison, 43 percent of Americans ate away from home for just over 40 percent of daily calories and fat. Given the prevalence of two career families, the lack of time available for home cooking, and the wide variety of choices available for meals away from home, the increase is not surprising".[41]

The interesting thing is until the 1990's less than 5% of the cases of childhood type 2 diabetes were seen by physicians, however, by 1994 and recently the rate has increased from 30 to 50% of all the type 2 diabetes cases. This increase inspired "Diabetes Care" to publish an article entitled "Emerging Epidemic of Type 2 Diabetes in Youth" where they looked at the increase in childhood and adolescent type 2 diabetes and its relationship to food intake. They cited a Japanese study of school children who were seven times more likely to have type 2 diabetes than type 1, which has increased 30 fold over the past 20 years connecting it to their eating habits and an increase in obesity rate.[42] The authors concluded by stating "the full effect of this epidemic will be felt as these children become adults and develop the long-term complications of diabetes."

At every turn, young people are targets for the unhealthy eating with very little consideration for their health. For instance, the school vending machine filled with junk food and fast foods sold to children on a minute-by-minute basis are mostly filled with food that have little to no nutritional values. A District of Columbia school inspector was reprimanded by elected public officials after he publicly criticized a school principal for promoting and selling junk and fast food on the school's grounds.[43]

With the frequency increasing of eating junk, fast, denatured, greasy foods, the population is becoming increasingly overweight, obese and diabetic because of lack of nutrients. Even though diabetes is to some extent considered a family genetic disease, it is mainly a consumptions disorder that impedes digestion causing an interruption of the balance between insulin, blood cells, food and glucose flow. This world culprit is lack of proper food combining along with the ingesting of bleached, refined, processed, greasy, overcooked foods, laced with harmful chemicals and striped of all their nutrients. The bleaching process of flour eliminates the bran and germ of wheat, leaving only white flour containing alloxan a chemical substance which has shown to cause diabetes in animals.[v,44] These foods lack fiber and enzymes altering the molecular structure of food, resulting in mal-absorption, introducing malnutrition, and resulting in overweight and obesity.

---

[v] Alloxan is the uric acid derivative initiates free radical damage to DNA in the beta cell of the pancreas, causing it to malfunction and die, Dr. Hari Sharma arthor of Freedom from Disease; The Enzyme Cure

These denatured foods cause the nutritional deficiencies that are related to diabetes and other health disparities. Processing removes vital nutrients from the food and aids food manufactures in the development of two or more food products from the same source. "Refining splits the whole grain into bran, germ, and endosperm, and it also removes all but the endosperm, which is the kernel's starchy center, added Dr. Walter Willett professor of epidemiology and nutrition, Harvard School of Public Heath, Boston, Mass. He went on to state "Ground fine, the endosperm is converted into flour that makes light and airy white bread, while the bran and germ are segregated to use in bran muffins and mixed into heavier breads that most Americans avoid." [45] These are some of the same foods diabetic are directed towards as part of their 4 to 6 small meals a day to maintain their blood sugar levels or foods to quietly increase their blood sugar levels when low. The impact of these foods increase the negative influence on the body's ability to heal from the diabetes.

There are several studies indentifying the relationship between food consumption and nutritional deficiencies as major contributing factors of type 2 diabetes. Dr. Willett conducted a 6 year study examining the role refined carbohydrates play in manifesting nutritional deficiencies of diabetes. In his study more than 65,000 women participated by consuming high amounts of carbohydrates in the form of white bread, potatoes, white rice, and pasta. These women had a two-and half times greater risk factors for type 2 diabetes than women in the study who consumed whole grain bread, and pasta. Because of this study, Dr. Willett suggested a reclassification of white bread and potatoes on the food pyramid, changing these foods to the category of sweet foods because they metabolize the same as sugar.[46]

The Iowa Women's Health Study, the Nurses' Health Study, and the Health Professionals Follow-Up Study tracked the health and dietary habits of 160,000 women over an 18 year period. They found women who consumed at least three servings of whole grains a day had a 20 to 30% lower risk of diabetes than women who consumed only one serving a week. [47]

The cover story in the May 2007 issue of the Nutrition Action Health letter, entitled "Whole Grains—The Inside Story" discuses 13 key elements lost in the refining process of whole grains and their link to diabetes. There is a 7% loss of vitamin E, 13% loss of B-6 and 16% of the magnesium is lost during milling of whole grain. Each one of these elements is important in the prevention of diabetes. In the article Joanne Slavin of the University of Minnesota stated, "We get too little exercise and eat too much high-calorie food. Our diet is broken, and you can't fix it by adding a few grams of whole grains or fiber." Ms. Slavin is referring to the process where manufacture strips the nutrients from grains and synthetically adds them back into the food calling them "Enriched". In the same article Alice Licthtenstein of Tufts University comments on the fact that 100% Whole Grain Chips Ahoy cookies worries her because it may send a signal to people increasing in take of cookies. She says "In a country where two out of three adults are overweight or obese, we eat too much of everything already.[48]

Grains stripped of nutrients are not the only foods contributing to diabetes, obesity, cardiovascular disease, high cholesterol and other disparities. Saturated fatty acids (lipids) are also an increasing threat. Lipids are fatty acids that the body needs for several hormonal processes. They maintain cell integrity and balance the immune system. However, when heated, lipids molecules change, creating saturated and trans-fatty acids, which increase adipose tissues development promoting unhealthy conditions relating to a high prevalence of overweight, obesity, diabetes and other health conditions. "According to modern pathology, or the study of disease process, an alteration in cell membrane function is the central factor in the development of virtually every disease. As it relates to diabetes, abnormal cell membrane structure due to eating the wrong types of fats leads to impaired action of insulin." commented Michael Murray, ND. He went on to state "The type of dietary fat profile linked to type 2 diabetes is an abundance of saturated fat and trans fatty acids (hydrogenated vegetable oils) along with a relative insufficiency of monounsaturated and omega 3 fatty acids." [49]

Ninety percent of type 2 diabetics are overweight or obese, which is a contributing factor of consuming the wrong type of fatty acids. The pancreas's beta cells depend on the proper function of fatty acids to maintain and increase insulin production in order to reduce blood glucose levels after a meal. The consumption of excessive saturated fatty acids disrupts the cells' ability to uptake glucose resulting in insulin resistance and type 2 diabetes. Studies of fatty acids' relationship to diabetes goes back as far as 1930 when H.P. Himsworth, MD, of the University College Hospital in London demonstrated how the habit of eating large quantities of fat increases glucose intolerance, compared to reversing the condition with carbohydrate-rich eating habits.[50]

The Making of Digestion; Absorption, Assimilation, and Elimination Problems in Glucose Control

"Currently, our country is facing an epidemic of digestive illness directly related to the foods we eat and the way we live. One-third to one-half of all adults have digestive illness-more than sixty-two million people."

Elizabeth Lipski, Ph.D., CNN Digestive Wellness

Food is a key element in the prevalence of type 2 diabetes, however, the most important factor is the ability to digest, absorb, assimilate nutrients and expel waste by products in a timely manner. In my research, I have not found information really identifying digestion, absorption and assimilation as a major contributing factor in the balance of blood sugar levels. Every article, book, journal or website I reviewed on diabetes hinted about the link of diabetes being a digestive (metabolic) disease however, no one ever came out and truly identified it as one in the sense of discussing the relative elements. There were no articles on the relationship between enzymes, proper food combining, digestion, absorption and assimilation. If medical science considered the above elements as the heart of diabetes and other diseases, they would understand how to heal these diseases rather than just treating the symptom. When dissecting diabetes, it shows a strong link is established between weight gain, improper eating habits, and a lack of exercise. This denotes a lack of digestion, absorption and assimilation establishing mal-absorption leading to malnutrition, which is a major part of diabetes. It also identifies the lack of the digestive enzymatic processing of foods, resulting in nutritional deficiencies of vital nutrients that increase weight gain, elevated glucose levels, and other complications surrounding diabetes.

Overweight and obese people carry around waste by products from undigested fast, fried, greasy, and denatured foods consumed lacking in enzymes. When the enzymatic process is reduced the body is unable to establish proper homeostasis. In the introduction of the book "Enzyme the Fountain of Life", it states, "Enzymes serve as the body's labor force to perform every single function required for our daily activities and required to keep us alive." It goes on to discuss, "In addition to our immune and defense systems, we require enzymes not only to eat, digest, and absorb our nutrients, but also to see, hear, smell, taste, breathe and move. [51] The pancreas is a major site of digestive enzymes needed to assist in proper digestion, absorption, assimilation and elimination.

There is no way we can not look at the pancreas and its enzymatic process in diabetes, because it is the major organ of distress. In fact, its function is not only to manufacture and secrete insulin, but also to promote enzymes to digest and absorb nutrients from the food. With diabetes this function is imparted resulting in excess glucose in the blood. The pancreas is responsible for degrading carbohydrates, lipids and sugars by the enzyme secretion process of amylase, sucrose and lipase. These processes occur in the mouth and small intestines where it chemically transforms starch into maltose to glucose, sucrose to glucose and fructose, lactose to glucose and galactose. [52]

Medical science has not investigated the link between overweight, obesity, diabetes, high cholesterol and other diseases with digestive enzymes. This process is essential for the nourishing of the body and maintaining the integrity of the body's systems and good health. The destruction begins with overcooked, processed, denatured and greasy foods lacking enzymes. They are either cooked out, processed or the food is harvested prematurely reducing nutritional values. For instance, bromelain is a protein degrading enzyme in fresh ripe pineapple, however, canned pineapple loss their valuable nutrients in the canning process.[53] When the food has no enzymes the body has to utilize its enzymes to digest the food reducing the body's supplements and increasing the risk of health conditions.[54] As a matter of fact, when looking at type 2 diabetes, it is orchestrated by weight gain and obesity, which is a direct result of foods not properly digesting, absorbing and assimilating to provide nourishment. The elements of food accumulate in the small intestine creates leaky gut syndrome resulting in not only diabetes, but high Dysbiosis, elevated cholesterol, cardiovascular disease, and other disparities.

The metabolic disorder of diabetes constitutes a malfunction of the digestive tract, specifically the pancreas's inability to secrete digestive enzymes, indicating the lack of nutritional absorption from the foods consumed. This mal-absorption of nutrients represents the loss of vital nourishment resulting in multi-nutritional deficiencies. Mal-absorption leads to malnutrition of the cells, causing overweight conditions, obesity, and type 2 diabetes, which is a risk factor for blindness, cardiovascular disease, retinopathy, coma, neuropathy and a major contributor to non-trauma limb amputations in the United States. Other conditions related to the diabetes's malnutrition include ulcers, diverticulitis, irritable bowel syndrome (IBS), abdominal pain, constipation, diarrhea, and gallstones.[55] The National Hospitalization data suggests that diabetic patients may also be more prone than the general population to gastrointestinal infections, cancer of the liver and pancreas, gastritis and other stomach disorders, intestinal impaction, liver disease, pancreatitis, and hematomesis", cited James E. Everhart, MD in an article on digestive Diseases and Diabetes.

Not only are the nutritional deficiencies of diabetes gastrointestinal related, but it also causes the deficiency of many different vitamins and minerals including magnesium, chromium, vanadium, zinc, and essential fatty acids. A lack in these vital nutrients shows an increase in the need for nutrients to heal diabetes and other health complications.

David F. Horrobin, PhD, emphasizes in the journal "Diabetes", that diabetic's should take a full range of nutritional supplements especially chromium, vitamin C, B6, zinc and alpha-lipoic acid. Each micronutrient is complementary linked to other individual micronutrients creating an intricate system for absorption, assimilation and nourishment. Without this delicate balance of nutritional interactions a person is unable to receive a full capacity of nutrients the body needs to maintain health and longevity, resulting in an increased risk of diabetes (type 1 and 2) and other health disparities. [56]

Published by the National Institute of Diabetes and Digestive and Kidney Diseases the summary of Chapter 21 on Digestive Disease and

Diabetes, authored by James E. Everhart, MD, MPH says, "Reviews of published clinical and epidemiologic studies reveal that it is difficult to demonstrate that people with diabetes are at much higher risk of digestive conditions than the general population, even for well characterized syndromes such as diabetes gastorpathy and diabetic diarrhea. The article goes on to discuss the fact that people with diabetes also suffer from constipation and other gastrointestinal disorders, with a high risk of celiac disease, chronic liver and gallbladder diseases.[57] Medial literature shows an inconsistency in their classification of whether diabetes is a digestive disorder or is a symptom of another digestive disorder. At any rate National Institute of Diabetes and Digestive and Kidney Disease (NIDDK) are not confirming diabetes as a digestive disease. Dr. Everheart continues in the article to state "for each digestive disease the discussion is organized to address two issues: whether diabetic subjects are at greater risk than non-diabetic subjects, and what characterizes the minority of diabetic people who develop the digestive diseases.[58] Despite the confliction of medical literature, diabetes is a digestive disorder of the entire alimentary tract with the pancreas as the major organ of interest. When the discussion surrounds diabetes's association with constipation, irritable bowel syndrome (IBS), diverticulitis, ulcers, abdominal pain, diarrhea, and gallstones, there is a direct connection having to do with the ability of the food to be digested, absorbed and assimilated properly in the body and not stored. The storage of food by product is what creates health issues.

As part of the digestive system the pancreas secretes enzyme into the small intestine to break down starches and carbohydrates with the enzyme amylase to simple sugars known as disaccharides. Trypsin is the enzyme that splits proteins into peptides small chains amino acids and lipase breaks down fats into fatty acids, all of which determines how our body is nourished and if the foods consumed remain in the intestinal tract longer then necessary. Once these elements are broken down the body is able to assimilate them and use them for energy, building blocks, and other functions to maintain health. When the pancreas is unable to work efficiently the body's energy is the first to suffer and the energy levels drop, creating tiredness sweet craven and in some cases weight gain. Weight gain is a primary issue of type 2 diabetes because the foods are not digesting and are accumulating in the small intestine where they are continuously decomposing.

A large percentage of diabetics, especially type 2 diabetics, suffer from constipation due to mal-absorption of nutrients. If we look at it constipation as a major aliment that is not classified as a disease, but is the major contributor of many disease. We spend over 75 billion dollars a year on laxatives to keep our bowels regular. The pancreas is connected to the small intestines where it secrets enzymes to assist in digestion, absorption and assimilation of nutrients from the foods consumed. When the pancreas is unable to complete this process, then the small intestines can't absorb and assimilate the nutrients in order for nourishment to take place. The waste by product store their self in the lining of the small intestine reducing its' ability to assimilate nutrients, instead it promotes waste into the blood stream, which is referred to as the Leaky Gut Syndrome.

The Leaky Gut Syndrome is an autoimmune deficiency syndrome where the foods consumed passes into the small intestine and accumulates there creating a toxic environment to the point the lining of the small intestine become irritated and the accumulated waste begins to leak into the blood stream. [59] When this waste leaks into the blood and the abdomen becomes distended (large) the blood becomes full of waste by products promoting other complications like high blood pressure, elevated cholesterol, cardiovascular disease, etc.; not to mention the diabetes issues of blindness and limb amputation. The gut flora is a major part of the immune system because of its ability to transport nutrients to nourish the body and keep it healthy. The gut is full of bacteria, most of which are healthy and needed; however, we destroy their ability to protect the body by consuming unhealthy products, antibiotics and other types of medicines. This is one of the causes of type 1 diabetes, where the immune system destroys the beta and alpha cells of the pancreas. This is very obvious in small children and infants who are given cow's milk or soy formulas and develop diabetes. The casein protein in the cow's milk disrupts the gut flora and reduces the ability of the gut to distribute nutrients through the body and protect the pancreas from destruction creating mal-absorption, and malnutrition.

The consumption of white flour product, white sugar, overcooked and greasy, fast foods, soda, processed foods, and consuming the wrong combination also destroys the gut flora food. All of these things contribute to the imbalance of the gut and creates problems with bowel illnesses such as celiac disease. Celiac disease shows up in type 1 diabetes after gluten is introduced to young children as diarrhea, malnutrition and weight loss. Constipation is also part of this illness as I have stated earlier. It is interesting that during my research I have not found much information linking bowel illnesses with diabetes, yet diabetes is classified as a digestive disease. Over the years of providing successful diabetes protocols I have witnessed changes in client's diabetes when they improved their lifestyle with good quality foods that increased nutrients that promoted their bowels without the use of laxatives. These nutrients promoted a frequency of bowels reducing and/or eliminating overweight conditions, obesity and diabetes. Again there is no hardcore research on bowels and diabetes; however, studies show when a diabetic increases their intake of fiber it reduces elevated blood glucose levels. The fiber creates a slower absorption of carbohydrates or sugar in the blood stream reducing the elevation of glucose in the blood and increases bowel movements. In order to fully understand the process you have to know the works of the digestive system. When discussing diabetes you can miss this as so many authors do. It is the key to reversing diabetes, because when the body is nourished there is no room for mal-absorption that leads to malnutrition.

The bowels are very important in any disease, especially one where the body is unable to receive nutrients like diabetes. One of the key elements in healing and reversing diabetes is eating good quality of foods with a high quality of absorbable vital nutrients. These foods would allow a free flow of the bowels reducing the time the waste remains in the intestinal tract leaking into the blood stream. One of the major causes is the consumption of foods that are almost indigestible by humans. Humans are not by nature carnivorous animals. We are herbivores (grass eaters) however; over the centuries humans have cultivated ourselves to consume meat products. There are several things that clearly demonstrate the types of food we need to eat to maintain health and longevity. Humans should eat fruits, grasses (grain), and vegetables and not meat, because it is indigestible in our intestinal system. Our intestinal system is 12 times our body size, where carnivorous animals' intestinal system are only 3 times the length of their body, making it a rapid system for the body to reduce the food, extract the nutrients and expel the waste by products in a timely manner. To also legitimize my discussion, one must consider their placement of the front teeth. Their front teeth are sharp and pointed to rip and tear the flesh apart because their do not chew their food; they gulp it down and have strong enough acid in their stomach break the meat down. The other interesting thing about carnivorous animals is how they eat meat raw to allow the enzyme cathepsin to break down the flesh. **I strongly do not advocate anyone eating raw meat.**

Humans do not possess the teeth or the acids needed to break down the flesh of meat. The fibers in the flesh are not digestible by humans even through we gulp our food like lower animals. When we gulp food it remains in the intestinal system for an extended period of time resulting in health issues, especially overweight conditions. Many people who have heard me speak on this subject have heard me say there are no fat people in the world; there are just people who are full of waste. This is the accumulation of waste byproducts from the undigested foods sitting in the intestinal system fermenting, putrefying and leaking into the blood stream. In her book, "Reversing Diabetes", Dr Whitaker states, "Our bodies are not designed to handle a lot of meat. While the first humans, without tools or weapons, would have had trouble acquiring much meat, carnivores are ideally suited for such. They have exceptionally strong jaws with sharp pointed fangs to kill other animals and tear their flesh into chunks that can be swallowed, as these animals do not chew their food, but swallow it whole."[60] She continues by addressing the fact that humans and carnivorous animals have significantly different digestive systems, with the hydrochloric acid of the carnivorous animal being twenty times greater then that of the fruit eater (human, vegetarian animals). She also compares the intestinal system between the two groups, stating "In addition, the intestinal tract of the meat eater is much shorter than that of the fruit eater-about four times the length of his body trunk as measured from the hips to the shoulders. For a meat eater the size of man, with a distance from hips to shoulders measuring about four feet, the intestinal tract would be about sixteen feet long. [61]

As Dr. Whitaker points out, the grass eaters do not have the intestinal system to consume meat products. The other point here is human have flat teeth that are not for tearing but for grinding the fruits, grains and leaves to be able to chew them well and receive vital nutrients from them. It enables humans to promote the proper enzyme to assist in the digestive process in order to absorb the nutrients and assimilate them into the body for health and well being. This is why it is important to understand the process of eating. Foods are the determining factor of how well the body will be and which type of disease a person will have or won't have.

One would ask the question, "If we are fruit, grain, and leaf eaters then why is it that diabetics can't eat fruits and lots of grains"? The answer is very simple, we have been cultivated to consume the wrong types of foods that have placed a hardship on the digestive system and the pancreas creating this imbalance promoting diabetes. We eat the wrong types of fruits and grains together, not digesting properly and thus increasing blood sugar levels. Over the past 2,000 or 3,000 years the food chain has evolved to where the food today is more unfit to eat then any other time in the history of the planet. Even through the Egyptians and people of other times had diabetes, it was not because their food had poor quality, it was for several other reasons.

During ancient times a system of eating together was a daily ritual. People sat and enjoyed their meal and combined the food in a way that was digestible. In today's world we eat too fast, almost never at the table as a family, always on the run, with all different kinds of combinations and foods laced with all types of additives, preservatives and dyes to make the food attractive.

In my research I have not come across any direct studies linking additives and preservatives to diabetes, however, one would suspect there is a relationship because the unnatural process of these chemicals has some bearing on the body's ability to function properly. We have to always remember that the body is a chemistry factory and when the wrong chemicals are mixed together they can create an explosion. The explosions we are witnessing are diabetes, obesity, cardiovascular disease, strokes and other health conditions that are also associated with diabetes. We have to seriously look at what is the chemical relationship between foods, the body and types of illness linked to diabetes.

The link to diabetes could very well be the fact that these chemical products are not digested in the body, but are being stored in the adipose tissues assisting in weight gain that is prevalent to type 2 diabetes. The testing and research needed for many of the additives and preservatives in the food and their link to diabetes and other illness are not being performed by the proper agencies. This is not only a health issue, but also a safety issue that somewhere down the line will have to be addressed. In the book, "Modern Foods: The Sabotage of Earth's Food Supply", there is a passage by Paul Sitt stating that " An ever-increasing proportion of the food we eat is no longer even food but is now a conglomerate of high-priced chemistry experiments designed to stimulate food. There are even chemicals like . . . Merlinerx, "The silly putty of the food world," which takes the place of the real thing in everything from cheese to brownies . . . Ruined natural ingredients, plus sugar, salt, fat and chemical additives. Put them all together and what do you get? You've got tantalizing phony foods that are high in refined carbohydrates and calories and devoid of nutritional value. It's a recipe for destruction-the formula for "Can't Eat Just One."[62] This statement sums up the discussion on the un-natural chemicals placed in the food. It also shows there is a nutritional issue when the chemistry of the food does not match the body, which results in mal-absorption, and malnutrition.

When we look at the situation of digestion, absorption, assimilation and elimination, we find that there are many factors to consider. I have only touched on a few but there are many more. For instance, when a person eats and is stressed out their digestive tract is up set and the digestive process is imbalanced, again resulting in mal-absorption. It is not just foods that create mal-absorption, but our emotional state has a great bearing on how well our food reacts to our body and whether we will receive nutrients from the food or not. This is another area where there is little to no research on the relationship between diabetes and emotions. There is information about how to ease your emotions when you have diabetes, but there is no link between emotions and mal-absorption of nutrients. For this I have to resort to my traditional Chinese background where diabetes is viewed very differently.

Digestion

Digestion is the chemical process of breaking down food into smaller particles that nourish the blood, tissues, cells, and organs. The digestive process determines how well food items are breaking down, absorbed, assimilated and how long it takes for the waste by products to be released. If for any reason the digestive process fails and the body is unable to receive nourishment, it may suffer from mal-absorption, resulting in mal-nutrition. Mal-absorption reduces the body's immunity, opening it up to a host of health conditions including malnutrition, which results in obesity, hypertension, diabetes, bowel problems, cancer and other unhealthy conditions.

Many of us grew up in family systems where it was not favorable to be thin. The saying "you need to put some meat on your bones". In today's world, being heavy (having some meat on your bones) indicates that the body is not digesting, absorbing and/or eliminating foods in a timely manner, resulting in overweight conditions that can cause other health conditions.

A child receives its first nutrients from its mother in the womb and immediately after through breastfeeding, which establishes their well-equipped digestive system. If the child is unable to receive the needed nutrients to support its body and immune system they will develop poor digestion that can last from birth to death. Improper digestion is an issue neither frequently addressed nor investigated by many health authors when researching obesity and other health conditions. Some researchers may mention the digestive system, however, it is not an in depth discussion. Perhaps the digestive system is not viewed as an important function to the life cycle process or perhaps society is more interested in counting calories; than understanding how food digest and if the calories are absorbed as nutrients that enhance the quality of the body's elements (blood, cells, tissues, organs, and systems).

The truth is digestion begins in the mind and not in the mouth. It begins with the sensory perceptions of smell, the way food looks, or the conversation about food. These three subjects stimulate the flow of gastric juices from the mouth to the small and large intestine. Sensory stimulation produces salivation in the mouth, churning the gastric juices in the stomach and the movement of peristalsis (motion that move the waste) in the colon. The mere smell of food can create rumbling in the intestinal tract; the rumbling sound of digestive juices churning sometimes cause abdominal discomfort. We refer to the churning as hunger pains. This sensation causes us to seek out some food to comfort us. We will then consume food to reduce the feeling of hunger. Once the food is consumed, the body has to determine what the food is before it can properly degrade it into useable nutrients. If the body is not able to determine the type of substances ingested, it will then turn the compounds of the food into waste (fermentation and putrefaction), in the small intestine where it turns into toxic waste that has the ability to leak into the blood creating all types of health conditions and maybe even death.

The chemical process for proper digestion includes elements such as enzymatic functions and hydrochloric acid process to separate and to assimilate minerals, vitamins, amino acids, proteins, carbohydrates, water, fats, antioxidants and other organic substances from food. Digestion is a basis for all chemical processes in the body through metabolism.

Metabolism further divides into Catabolism and Anabolism. The mechanism by which food particles are metabolized (broken down) from large particles to smaller ones and released, as energy is known as Catabolism. On the other hand, the uptake of energy from the food particles is an Anabolism reaction promoting the energy movement creating digestion, circulation, respiration and other bodily functions. Metabolism converts food into energy. This energy turns into blood, cells, tissues, organs and body fluids, without which there would be no living organism. The health of the body depends on whether the metabolic process is able to use the food as energy and be able to eliminate the waste by products from the body in a timely manner. When wastes by products are allowed to accumulate in the small intestine for a matter of time it breeds unhealthy bacteria that increase the prevalence of disorders (elevated cholesterol, hypertension, overweight and obesity, etc).

Once again, the process of digestion does not begin in the mouth it begins in the mind. The sight, smell or discussion of food, stimulate the olfactory nerve, which promotes digestive juices to flow, inducing the feeling to consume food or beverages. Taste, on the other hand, occurs when food is placed in the mouth by the tongue sensory cells. Each area of the tongue has different sensory cells for specific tastes.

Many food-processing companies add dye and preservatives to foods in order to make it look, smell and taste appealing. Food manufactures know when a person comes in contact with food products, it will stimulate a chemical reaction in the body triggering craving for that product. In some conditions, consumers can become addicted to the product (coffee, sugar, etc.) because after ingesting the product a few times the body becomes dependant on the food, especially if the food is sweet (there is a very high sweet craven amongst the US population. If there was research done on this factor, it may come out to 3 out of 5 people crave sweets on a daily basis.)

Gastrointestinal Tract

As we know diabetes is a multi-digestive disorder, making the digestive tract a major contributor to the disease. By understanding the process of digestion you will have a better knowledge of how to address diabetes and how the use of minerals, vitamins, herbs and other nutrients will interact with the body and work to revere diabetes. This information increases your knowledge of how to improve the immune system, which is a large part of your digestive tract working to maintain immunity. Your immunity is depended on your bodies' ability to digest, absorb, and assimilate nutrients from foods consumed, as it expels waste byproduct in a timely manner. When this does not occur the body systems become backed up and the immune system is not able to protect the body.

The digestive system consists of the gastrointestinal tract, which is a 29.5 foot long tubular muscle that starts from the mouth to the anus and is the major carrier of food through the gastrointestinal tract. The tract consists of smooth muscle and connective tissue on the outer layer. The inner layer consists of epithelium mucous membranes (mucosa), which secrets mucus to protect the gastrointestinal tract, as well as enzyme secreting glands to digest food molecules into usable energy and nutrients.

There are two inner layers of the gastrointestinal tract, the sub mucosa and the serous levels are comprised of smooth muscle creating contractions with in the gastrointestinal tract. One set of muscle wrap around the gastrointestinal tract and cause the tract to decrease in diameter developing the peristaltic movement of the gastrointestinal tract. The other muscles is the entire length of the gastrointestinal tract causing the tract to contract by way of shortening and lengthening the tract as it also promotes parasitical movements. The sub mucosa level is comprised of blood vessels, nerve tissues, lymphatic vessels and carries away absorbed material.

Digestive Processes

The Mouth

After one has consumed food, the food enters the oral cavity consisting of the mouth, tongue, teeth, lips, cheeks, hard and soft palates. The mouth is where food is chewed (masticated), by the teeth and mixed with saliva by the tongue, which is connected to the floor of the mouth by the frenulum, (a fold of tissue) where the food is transformed into a liquid bolus and swallowed. The tongue is comprised of the taste buds (papillae), skeletal muscle that is covered by mucus membrane. Food is then mixed with starch and digestive enzymes before swallowed. When this process is obstructed or inhibited by a lack of chewing or drinking, the body becomes unable to receive nourishment from food.

The mouth houses the teeth, which consist of the 20 deciduous (baby teeth) that are shed in childhood. When we lose the childhood teeth they are replaced by 32 permanent teeth. The four classifications of adult teeth are the incisors, which are in the front of the mouth; they are used to bite off pieces of food. The cones shaped cuspids (canines) are for tearing and grasping food. The third set of the teeth found in the back of the mouth are the bicuspids (premolars) and molars, which are both flat and used to grind the food.

The mouth is an alkaline environment; the tongue houses the sensory receptors taste buds stimulating chemical reaction to digest starch through an enzyme called amylase. The mouth receptors identify taste (sour, bitter, pungent, sweet, salty), texture, and temperature of foods to be digested. However, the body can be fooled by the incorrect combination of food. The results of these incorrect combinations can cause indigestion, gas, constipation, gastric reflex and other gastrointestinal illness.

Salivary glands play a major role in the digestive process, without the salivary glands there would be no lubrication in the mouth. Each of the three sets of salivary glands (parotid, sub mandibular or sub maxillary), are sublingual glands which aid in the degrading of starch by the secretion of enzyme amylase. There will be more information about amylase in the discussion on enzymes.

The hard palate is the roof of the mouth it begins in the front and extends to the back of the mouth where it intersects with the soft palate. The soft palate houses the uvula, a cone shape projection in the mouth. The soft palate also houses the palatine tonsils and pharyngeal tonsils (adenoids), which are lymphatic tissue.

Once you have masticated the food well, then the bolus is ready to enter the esophagus where it will move to the stomach. The esophagus is a 10-inch long straight collapsible, muscular tube that passes through the diaphragm where food passes from the mouth to the stomach. This passing of food has to do with deglutition (swallowing) and coordination of the tongue, soft palate, esophagus and pharynx functions. This process causes the esophagus to contract crating peristalsis, which is a wave like motion that moves the bolus along until it reaches the cardiac sphincter where it enters the stomach.

The Stomach

Food leaves the mouth and travels down the esophagus into the stomach. This C shaped organ is anatomically positioned in the upper left hand quadrant of the abdomen. It's comprised of the cardia, fundus, and pylorus. The internal lining of the stomach contains the rugae, which are folds in the lining that are more obvious when the stomach is not distended.

The stomach stores food in an acidic environment where hydrochloric acid along with pepsin the major digesting enzyme breaks down protein. The nitrogen base of protein (more on protein components in a later session) gives it a composition that has to be degraded in an acid environment. The stomach secretes mucus to protect the lining of the stomach from the harsh hydrochloric acid.

There is what is known as the intrinsic factor of the stomach, this factor aligns itself with B12 in order to guide it through the hydrochloric acid to the alkaline small intestines where it is absorbed. Most people have insufficient stomach intrinsic factor, which is the reason B12 has to be introduced with other vitamins, intravenous injected or taken sublingual (under the tongue). The stomach also absorbs small amounts of other elements such as alcohol, ions, glucose and water.

The production of pepsinogen, which is the precursor of pepsin is produced and regulated by the hormonal gastrin in the stomach. Gastrin is also responsible for the regulation of hydrochloric acid and mucus in the stomach. As the stomach churns, it reduces the undigested food to chyme that is moved through the pyloric sphincter by peristaltic action (wave like movement) into the small intestine where the majority of assimilation and absorption takes place. When the acid environment of the stomach functions improperly, proteins will not digest and moves into the alkaline environment of the small intestine where it putrefies. If the protein is unable to digest in the stomach, it could cause other types of problems such as reflex, indigestion, heartburn, etc.

When a person drinks an abundance of any liquid whether hot or cold at the same time they consume food it alters the digestive juice balance, (especially hydrochloric acid) hindering the digestive process. When the liquid is cold, it really affects the hydrochloric acid's temperature and disrupts the ability to digest proteins. It is not advisable to drink while eating a meal. Fluids should be consumed an hour before or an hour after a meal. The only time a person should drink at the time of eating is when taking supplements, and only enough water should be consumed to swallow the supplement. The only other time one should drink and eat is when consuming bulky fibrous foods like brain, psyllium, etc.

Protein should always be eaten by it self, it makes it easier to digest. Another thing to remember is that starch will not digest in the stomach because it needs an alkaline environment for digestion. Starches will only ferments in the stomach.

Small Intestine

The small intestine is an alkaline environment that is the most important organ of digestion, because it is the site of absorption and assimilation of nutrients or it supplies the blood with waste in the leaky gut syndrome. As food leaves the stomach, it enters the first 12 inches of the small intestines by way of the duodenum. The extension of the small intestine is from the duodenum to the ileocecal sphincter a circular muscle in the abdomen and pelvis. There is also a valve at the point of the ileocecal that sometimes clogs causing abdominal pain. When clogged it prevents food from passing to the large intestine. The duodenum is where the chyme comes in contact with bicarbonates ions that transformed the acid pH of the chyme into an alkaline substance.

This alkaline environment of the small intestine provides the ability of enzyme to digest and degrade the food particle in the chyme, allowing it to release nutrients for absorption in the jejunum and ileum. The duodenum is where the majority of digestion occurs. At the site of the duodenum, is the lumen where enzymes enter through glands of the crypt or crypts of lieberkuha, which are pits in the intestine. The Peyer's patches of the submucosa as part of the lymphatic system and also contains the alkaline secreting mucus glands called Brunners glands. The pancreas supplies enzymes that assist in the digestion of carbohydrates, sugars and fats.

The liver contributes to the small intestine's ability to absorb by the secretion of bile. The process is the liver manufactures bile and secretes it to the gallbladder, which stores it and secretes it through the common duct into the small intestines where it degrades fat globules and sugar.

Once the chyme is neutralized, transformed into an alkaline substance and digested by enzymes and the bile salts, it is ready for absorption and assimilation into the body. This occurs in the jejunum and ileum. The jejunum and ileum area of the small intestine performs very little digestion and more absorption with its finger like projections villi and microvilli of the mucosa. The membrane of the mucosal cells house microscopic microvilli projections. They are a rich series of capillaries and lacteals (lymphatic vessel) within the membrane walls of the villi. The digested product of carbohydrates, protein, and nucleic acid are found in the capillaries. On the other hand, products from the digestion of fat are founding the lacteals.

Absorption is a process for transformation of intestinal fluids through the epithelial cell walls of the small intestine, into the capillaries[vi] using adenosine triphosphate (ATP) and carrier molecules. The capillaries are also the site of electrolytes, water, and vitamin absorption into the blood. Amino acids, monosaccharide and short-chained fatty acids are absorbed through the blood capillaries. Long-chain fatty acids form triglycerides that are resyntherzied and undergo a process called diffusion, which occurs in order for the fatty acids to be absorbed into the lymphatic[vii] capillary (lacteals) of the small intestines. The small intestins is also the site of probiotics, healthy gut bacteria to support the immune system.

The Pancreas

The pancreas is an oblong gland that is one inch thick and five inches long. It is located in the center of the abdomen posterior to the great curvature of the stomach. It connects to the duodenum by two ducts, the pancreatic duct (duct of Wirsung) and the accessory duct (duct of Santorini). The Ampulla of Vater is the common meeting place for the duct of Wirsung and the common duct of the liver and gallbladder to enter the duodenum. The entrance of the duct of Santorini into the duodenum is about one inch above the Ampulla of Vater. The functional digestive cells that secrete pancreatic juice and provide the exocrine portion of the pancreas are the acini cells.

The pancreatic juices have slightly alkaline pH balance that neutralizes acid material for the stomach. These juices are colorless liquids containing bicarbonates, salts, water, and other elements for digestion. It provides several different enzymes to digest and degrade carbohydrates (amylase), lipids fats (lipease), ribonuclease, deoxyribonucleic, and nucleic acids, proteins. The hormone secretion and cholecystokinin are also controlled by the pancreas.

The Liver

The liver is the clearinghouse of the body and the largest gland in the body. It has a major role in gastrointestinal functions. It is engaged in performing over one hundred different functions, which allows it to

---

[vi] Capillary: Small blood vessel connecting arteriole and venule. Human Anatomy and Physiology; Brown Company Publishers

aid the body in maintaining health and well-being. When the liver is out of balance, the entire body is out of balance. It is located in the right hypochondrium of the upper abdomen cavity under the diaphragm. It is divided into four lobes consisting of the right, left, cordate and quadrate. Within these lobes are subdivisions called lobules, containing hepatocytes, and Kupffer cells, which are cells of the reticuloendothelial system.

The hepatic portal system of the liver receives nutrients and other substance that are absorbed by the digestive system. This process is carried out through the venules and veins that make up the hepatic portal that drains this material from the digestive system's capillaries. The hepatic artery provides the liver with material from the circulator system. The liver also releases material into the body for circulation by way of the hepatic vein.

The liver manufactures bile a yellow or olive-green liquid substance consisting of water, bile salts, cholesterol, lecithin (a phospholipids), bile pigments and several ion. Bilirubin, the pigment of bile is derived from the heme portion of the break down of red blood cells (hemoglobin). The intestinal bacteria latter digest Bilirubin, transferring it into other substance like urobilinogen, which is part of feces color.

After the liver produces bile, it's secretes it into the gallbladder where it is stored. The gallbladder is a pear-shaped sac that is located on the visceral surface of the liver, where it drains through the cystic duct into the duodenum through the common bile into the small intestine, aiding in the digestion of lipids (fats). The formulation of the common duct is from the cystic duct of the gallbladder and the hepatic duct of the liver.

The liver converts nutrients from food and gastrointestinal tract into new enriched blood. This blood is pumped from the liver through the vena cava (large vein) to the heart where it re-circulates fresh blood back into the body. Many sugars (starch, carbohydrates, sugar, honey, maple syrup, etc) are metabolized and transformed into glycogen by the liver, and then introduced into the system as glucose for energy. A healthy liver is able to except large doses of sugar from intestinal blood, and with enzyme convert the protein glycogen to glucose (the process is called glycogenolysis) causing blood glucose levels to rise. The affects of glycogen elevating blood sugar levels are sometimes referred to as *hyperglycemic factor*. This elevation ends when the body has enough sugar in the blood and it keeps the body from hypoglycemia (Low blood sugar). The transformation of glycogen is the direct opposite of insulin, which lowers the blood sugar levels. On the other hand if blood glucose levels are low, then the process of glycogenolysis is unable to occur where the liver enzymes transforms glycogen into glucose. Another process gluconeogenesis is when the liver converts amino acids into glucose.

The liver also degrades fatty acids into acetyl coenzyme A, which are further processed to release the energy of the chemical bond. Deamination of protein is another function of the livers in regards to metabolic process. Deamination is the process where the liver removes the nitrogen portion from the amino acids, which are converted into urea and excreted in the urine. This process can produce energy or it can convert this energy to carbohydrates or fat through its transformation of amino acids into an amino acid group, which synthesizes urea. The liver synthesizes other forms of protein, like plasma protein used in blood clotting (albumin, fibrinogen, globulins, and prothrombin). The liver is a storage depot for many nutrients such as vitamins A, B12, D (activates body usage), E, and K. Iron is a mineral that is also stored in the liver. The liver's kupffer cells promote phagocytes, where these cells eradicate red and white used blood cells and foreign material from the bloodstream.

Diseases of the Digestive Tract

As I have discussed the digestive tract, I will now identify some disease of the digestive tract only because some people with diabetes also find their self with some of these digestive disorders. The chart will identify the disorder, explain what it is, it's cause, symptoms and association. If as a diabetic you do not have any of these, than as diabetes prolongs in your life you may find your self with one or more of them and you will be able to identify them and their causes.

Disease name	What is it	Cause	Symptoms	Diseases association
Dysbiosis: Living together in mutual harmony	When the healthy micro flora of the intestines is disrupted.	High levels of stress, Toxic chemicals, (manufactured), devitalized food, oral	Bloating, abdominal discomfort, indigestion, constipation,	Rheumatoid arthritis, diabetes, ankylosis spondylitis, eczema,

		contraceptives, antibiotics, pain pills, non steroidal anti-inflammatory drugs, (NSAID's) and surgery.	diarrhea, fatigue, gas, irritable bowel syndrome,	psoriasis, allergies, leaky gut syndrome, connective tissue diseases, obesity,
Candida	Yeast and fugal infection of the intestine and the blood.	Antibiotic usage, consumption of an abundance of sugar, oral contraceptives, NSAID's.	Abdominal bloating, anxiety, constipation, diarrhea, depression, sensitivity to the environment, recurring bladder or vaginal infections, inability to concentrate, insomnia, moodiness, PMS, low blood pressure, sensitivity to smells, allergies,	Autoimmune disease, Malabsorption of nutrients, malnutrition
Leaky Gut Syndrome: Hyper-permeability	Toxins and bacteria's leak through the lining of the small intestine into the blood.	Candida, medications, alcohol, HIV, severe burns, chemotherapy, radiation, chemical additives, enzyme deficiencies, caffeine, parasites, contaminated food and water, dyes, preservatives, artificial flavoring, pesticides, free radicals, junk food, dental toxins, stress, antacids, antibiotics, steroids, NSID's,	Food allergies, chronic fatigue, hives, alopecia aerate,	multiple sclerosis, diabetes, thyroiditis, lupus, ulcerative colitis, chrone's disease, raynaud's disease, sjogren's syndrome fibromyalgia, rheumatoid arthritis, polymyalgia rheumatic,

Constipation	Infrequent bowel movement of hard stools. Bowel movements that are hard and inconsistent.	Improper consumption of foods including fried, greasy, processed, and over cooked foods and junk foods. Antibiotics (they remove the healthy bacteria from the colon). Dairy products, insuffent consumption of fiber, medications, improper abortion of iron supplements, inadequate exercise, inadequate consumption of water, long term laxative use.	Abdominal distention, allergies, fatigue, bloating, feeling of heaviness	High blood pressure, overweight/obesity, bad breath, diverticulitis, gas, headaches, indigestion, hemorrhoids, varicose veins, colon cancer.
Diarrhea				
Irritable Bowel Syndrome				

Diabetics have been known to have some of these bowel disorders at one time or another and in most case have not been documented or linked to diabetic condition.

In traditional Chinese medicine bowel issues are caused by either hot or cold, excessiveness, deficient or stagnation issues in the liver, spleen, stomach, small and/or large intestines. You will find more information about traditional Chinese medicine in chapters to come.

What's Cholesterol Got to Do With It

"A person cannot succeed in anything without a good, sound body-a body that is able to stand up against hardships, that is able to endure."

Booker T. Washington 1856-1915

High cholesterol is the second cousin to diabetes, in some cases it can be the cause of diabetes. Cholesterol is a needed element of the body. The Merck Manual of Medical Information states, "Cholesterol and triglycerides are important fats (lipids) in the blood."[63] Humans can't live without cholesterol because it is essential to everyday life. It comprises the cell membrane, the manufacturing of vitamin D a fat-soluble vitamin, formulating bile salts and hormones, as well as maintaining the development and integrity of nerve and brain cells. Through the function of the liver the body can manufacture a substantial amount of cholesterol high-density lipoproteins (HDL—good cholesterol) to sufficiently address the body's needs. The body also receives cholesterol for foods, some good cholesterol and some increases low-density lipoproteins (LDL—bad cholesterol).

Because of the incompatibility of fats and water, (which is the major composition of the blood), cholesterol and triglycerides are unable to freely circulate through the body without an aid. The aid is known as a lipoprotein. It is the merge between lipids (fat) and a protein that is surrounded by phospholipids and carried through the blood by apoproteins. Cholesterol is classified by its integrity in the body and how it performs in assisting the body to maintain health and well being. This classification is either high-density lipoproteins or very low and low-density lipoproteins. High-density lipoproteins (HDL) are in abundance in the body and assist in the production of healthy elements to maintain a healthy body. On the other hand, the very low and low-density lipoproteins are the destructive cholesterols and causes high blood pressure, cardiovascular disease, atherosclerosis, stroke and other life threatening diseases.

Most type 2 diabetics are found to have "high" low-density lipoproteins (LDL—bad cholesterol) and "low" high-density proteins (good cholesterol), making them at risk for heat attack, stroke and hypertension. In a study that appeared in Diabetes Care, where over a 2 year period Heinz Drexel, M.D. and colleagues at Vorarlberg Institute for Vascular Investigation and treatment and the Department of Medicine, Academic Teaching Hospital Feldrirch, Feldkirch, Austria, studied 750 patients undergoing coronary angiography. The study investigated three different groups of people, one group had normal fasting glucose levels, another had impaired and the third had type 2 diabetes. They found that low HDL's and high triglycerides were associated with hyperglycemia and Coronary Artery Disease in type 2 diabetics.[64]

High triglycerides and cholesterol are promoted through diabetics eating habits of greasy fried foods, high sugar intake that turn to fat and are stored in the body. There is no literature I have found to validate drinking liquids and eating at the same time as being a cause of high cholesterol and triglycerides, **but if you just visited digestion**, enzyme therapy and the consumption of food and drink you would see that there is a possibility that drinking and eating could cause cholesterol issues. When a person eats and drinks at the same time they reduce the enzymatic process of the body. In most cases the liquid is cold and the food is greasy which makes for the grease to become hard like lard, resulting in a waxy thick substance lodged in the arteries creating obstructions.

Medical science has not really investigated the role eating has on the body. They are just touching the surface. There needs to be more research on the interaction between food, drinking and eating at the same time. Over my 30 plus years in wholistic health care I have found that when a person eliminates drinking with a meal and only drink enough room temperature water to take supplements several things happen. They find their food digest different and easier, also their bowel movements change and they don't feel full after a meal, but very comfortable. They also find they don't gain weight, but lose it because their body is now processing the food and extracting the nutrients from the food. This also allows the enzymatic function to promote the separation of the nutrients from the waste by products and aid in frequent and healthy bowel movements.

I have also seen this process of not drinking and eating in conjunction with taking lecithin, a phospholipid to reduce and/or eliminate elevated cholesterol and high triglycerides in a matter of weeks. There were clients whose cholesterol was high and they began my protocol. Both my client and their physician were amazed at the result within weeks. I will discuss more on lecithin later. All I can say now is that if your cholesterol or triglycerides are high you need to rush out to the health food store and pick up some lecithin today. Vitamin B3 niacin has been shown in several studies to reduce elevated cholesterol. I recommend you take both lecithin and *non-flush* niacin together for best results.

Most of the time when we hear about cholesterol it is negative because of its connection to cardiovascular disease, obesity and other unhealthy conditions. Cholesterol is a natural element of all our body cell membrane, including bile and sterol hormone-like substances. Cholesterol is steroid lipid manufactured by the liver (1,000 MG a day) or from foods consumed and transported throughout the circulating blood of all animals. When fatty acids are ingested they convert to diglycerides and then to monoglycerides in order to be absorbed as free fatty acids. When absorbed free fatty acids connect to a protein they become lipoproteins and are transported throughout the body. We know these lipoproteins as very low-density lipoproteins (VDL), low-density lipoproteins (LDL) or high-density lipoproteins (HDL). They are best known for their cholesterol levels descriptions. The liver and gallbladder play a significant role in the ability of triglycerides digestion and absorption in the body because of the hormones they manufacture and secrete known as bile salts.

Cholesterol has its place not only in the blood plasma but 10% of the brains lipids are comprised of cholesterol. However, it can cause havoc when out of balance increasing the low-density lipoproteins (LDL) elevating cholesterol (bad) levels and endangering the body. Very low and low-density lipoproteins are what obstruct the arteries with plague resulting in heart attacks, strokes, hypertension and other degenerative diseases. On the other hand, high-density (good cholesterol) lipoproteins increase the flow of blood taking cholesterol back to the liver to be synthesized.

Cholesterol is a major part of the American's eating habit to the point where the average adult male consumes 337 milligrams and adult female consume 217 milligrams according to the American Heart Association. They recommend that the daily intake of cholesterol is below 160 milligrams a day. It is suggested that persons who have cardiovascular disease or other vascular health conditions should not exceed 100 milligrams of cholesterol a day. LDL is mainly the product of saturated fatty acids that are consumed from meats, lards, butters, and margarines. Low-density lipoproteins can also come from eating foods with large amounts of carbohydrate in the form of refined sugars.

The National Cholesterol Education Program guidelines for triglycerides are:

Normal	Less than 150 mg/dL
Borderline-high	150 to 199 mg/dL
High	200 to 499 mg/dL
Very high	500 mg/dL or higher

These are based on fasting plasma triglyceride levels.

This information is from the American Heart Association

Phospholipids have a structure similar to triglycerides however; they are different in their constituent because they are the primary matrix of the cell membrane, balancing water and lipid interchange within cell membranes. Phospholipids comprise cell membranes with the brain containing 35 percent, the eyes account for 60 percent of the DHA (docosahexaenoic acid) omega 3 fatty acid.[65] In the book "Clinical Nutrition a Functional Approach," it states "Especially in developing infants, changes in DHA composition in nervous system tissue have been suggested as contributor to such conditions as attention deficit and hyperactivity disorder and may influence visual capacity."[66]

Lecithin

"What does it mean to "eat from the place of spirit?" It would mean being "present with your eating," says Dr. Mayer, "and not taking food for granted. Every single taste in the food would be more appreciated."

Deborah Kesten
Feeding the Body Nourishing the Soul

Lecithin, with the composition as phosphatidyl choline, plays a major role in the balancing of phospholipids present in cells.[67] When a person eats healthy their liver will produce lecithin, which is the building block of cellular membranes. It is the primary substance maintaining homeostasis of cell membranes. The brain and the brain stem are unable to function without a significant amount of lecithin.[68] Lecithin is also a fat emulsifier and has the ability to reduce cholesterol levels in blood and blood vessels.[69] It can also be taken as a supplement and is found in liquid and pill form in all health food stores and some major grocery stores. It is processed from either egg yolks or soybeans. Because of the increase of allergic reactions to soya it is best to consume lecithin from eggs.

Micronutrient Deficiencies Associated to Diabetes

"The power of nature to cure itself, and thus the belief that there was a natural tendency for things to get better on their own. This tendency could be aided by providing a beneficial environment for the patient and by improving physical function with a regiment of suitable diet and exercises."

Medicine A History of Healing

The minerals, vitamins, amino acids and other trace elements that should be in the food are what aids in maintaining the health of the body. When these elements are lacking in the foods and these elements are not supplemented, the body begins to rapidly decompose. Diabetes is classified as a wasting disease; meaning the cellular structure of the body is unable to regenerate it's self and is not able to maintain its own integrity. This is why over time some diabetics become blind, require limb amputation and suffer with other complications.

All foods have some type of nutrient that will support life. When we study lower animals we find they consume only the foods that provide them with the best nutrients. They basically do not eat out of their nutritional range unless we domesticate them and teach them to eat what we eat. When they receive the proper nutrients they normally die of natural causes at the proper time and not premature death as humans do.

Studies show that diabetes is a disease of nutritional mal-absorption; a lack of vital nutrients to support the body's daily functions. They also indicate that replacing the nutrients can reverse diabetes. As society continues to promote the movement of Functional Medicine, we begin to witness the growth of many different health conditions that are nutritional related and diabetes is one.

In an article published by the Albion Research Notes states, "The nutritional emphasis of traditional medical management of diabetes has revolved around macronutrient intake. In fact, a quick glance at recent medical and nutritional texts on the subject show that established medical opinion is that diabetics have the same micronutrient needs as non-diabetic."[70] This statement works to compare diabetics nutritional values to be equal with non diabetics, however, in the article's next statement it contradicts itself by stating, "In reviewing clinical studies published on this topic over the last few years, it becomes apparent that several minerals are of great importance and have potential impact on the typical diabetic individual."[71] The author demonstrates the medical community has knowledge of links between micronutrients deficiencies and diabetes even through they prefer to use drugs and not nutrients to invigorate the bodies ability to heal it self from diabetes. They look to suppress the disease, instead of healing the body from the disease. In the article certain minerals were identified as being deficient in diabetics including magnesium, zinc, chromium, manganese, copper and selenium. The article equated the excessive loss of these vital minerals to diabetic polyuria[viii] one of the major cause of nutritional losses.[72]

Chromium

A nutritional deficiency of chromium results from the consumption of refined foods causing hyperglocimumia (diabetes mellitus) or immune deficiencies as in type 1 diabetes.[73] Chromium has been sited in numerous studies for its ability to improve insulin sensitivity, lower blood glucose levels, reduce low density lipoprotein (LDL), and increase high density lipoprotein activity.[74] Chromium is an essential mineral in the metabolic process working with insulin to promote glucose transition from blood to cell. In its role, chromium assists in reducing plaque build up in the arteries, reducing diabetic's risk of arteriosclerosis. There are

---

[viii] Polyuria is a condition characterized by the passage of large volumes of urine (2.5Liters over 24 hours in adults), frequent urination: Wikipedia The Free Encyclopedia

some studies indicating no real change in glucose levels with chromium, however, according to Richard A. Anderson, Ph.D., "the inability of chromium to reduce blood glucose levels is due to using dosage of 200 mgc or less. These low dosages are in adequate for diabetics because of their low absorption rate."[75] In his research, Anderson and colleagues divided 180 type 2 diabetics into three groups where they administered chromium in dosages of 200 mcg/day to one group, 1,000 mcg/day to another and a placebo group. Their finding after 2 months showed the higher dosages group had significant improvement in their glycosylated hemoglobin. They noticed after 4 months of therapy both chromium groups had significant improvement in their glycosylated hemoglobin. The improved glycosylated[ix] hemoglobin showed an average of 6.6% in the high-dose group, 7.5% in the low dose group and 8.5% in the placebo group after 4 months. The high dosages of chromium improved the fasting blood sugar and 2 hours after-eating insulin levels.[76] Chromium is an important trace mineral in the glucose tolerance factor (GTF), which involves a binding of chromium, niacin, glycine, glutamic acid, and cysteine. Chromium is a vital asset assisting insulin in facilitating the assimilations of glucose into cells.

The body uses chromium to metabolize carbohydrates, lipids and to increase insulin's activity in a manner that it reduces and maintains positive blood sugar levels. One of the many ways our body loses chromium is through kidney secretions in the urine. It is a major part of the glucose tolerance factor (GTF), which contains niacin (B_3), glycine, glutamic acid, cysteine and chromium. There is a synergistic relationship between chromium and vanadium when consumed together. They lower blood sugar levels, regulate blood vessels and reduce elevated cholesterol. However, chromium by it self can improve LDL levels. Many expecting mothers find themselves with gestational diabetes because the fetus is extracting much of the chromium.[77] Chromium absorbs easier when taken in the Picolinated form, which is a natural occurring amino acid metabolite. The average Western eating habit is deficient in chromium because of it's destruction during food processing. Sugary foods tend to deplete chromium in the body and we don't consume enough foods containing chromium for us to build it in our body to ward off hypoglycemia or elevated cholesterol.

[ix] Glycosyland forms a glycoprotein by adding a glyocsyl group (sugar) to a protein. Merriam Webster's Medical Desk Dictionary.

Food Sources:

Asparagus, barley, beer, black pepper, blackstrap molasses, brewer's yeast, broccoli, brown rice, cheese, chicken, clams, corn and it's oil, dulse (seaweed), egg yolks, grapes, honey, legumes, meat, mushrooms, nuts, oysters, potatoes, raisins, rhubarb, seeds, wheat cereals, whole grain and wine.

RDA Children 10-60 mcg   Adults 50-200 mcg

Absorption contributors: Chromium is easier to be absorbed by the body with copper, iron, manganese zinc.

Inhibitors: aluminum cookware, all white sugar proudcts

Taken in the supplemental form there is caution because it will lower blood sugar levels, so the blood sugar should be checked often to make sure the levels do not drop too low. The daily recommended requirement is 200 to 350 mcg a day.

Magnesium

Several studies have revealed that diabetics need twice the amount of magnesium than their non-diabetic counterparts, which is linked to retinopathy.[78] Magnesium deficiencies have shown to be related to alteration of glucose metabolism, cardiac arrhythmias, high blood pressure, and myocardial infraction (heart attack). According to Dr. Robert K. Rude of the University of California, School of Medicine at Los Angeles. Dr Rude states, "Actually, the association between low magnesium levels and diabetes has been documented since 1946. Insulin may enhance magnesium transport into the cells, and therefore, insulin resistance may result in intracellular magnesium deficit." He goes on to explain, that magnesium supplementation either intravenously or orally will have an impact on reducing the risk of complication for people who are diabetics or people taking diuretics.[79] Magnesium plays a vital role not only in the development of DNA and RNA, but also in the conversion of carbohydrates, proteins and fats for the body to use as energy and reduce the levels of glucose in the blood. Magnesium is required for both proper glucose utilization and insulin signaling.

Metabolic alterations in cellular magnesium, which may play the role of a second messenger for insulin action, contribute to insulin resistance, is the conclusion of an article published in the Metabolic Research Journal entitled Intercellular Magnesium and Insulin Resistance.[80]

Magnesium interaction with other nutrients is vital for the process of absorption and assimilation. When magnesium is deficient it creates absorption and assimilation issues with nutrients such as calcium, phosphorus, protein, vitamin C, D, and B complex especially B 6, 12, and fat synthesizing, according to Donald J. Lepore, ND, DN, NMD.[81] In addition, the deficiency of magnesium impairs the body's ability to properly manufacture lecithin, allowing cholesterol levels to elevate, increasing the risk of cardiovascular disease in type 2 diabetics. Every living cell in the body has lecithin to aid in the digestion, and absorption of lipids. Lecithin's emulsifying activity degrades lipids into tiny droplets that allow the lipids to be assimilated through the small intestine into the cells as it reduces cholesterol and fatty acids in the body. It is the natural substance in the myelin sheath protective covering of the nerves.[82]

When magnesium is deficient it reduces the uptake of potassium and calcium creating other mineral deficiency. Magnesium is known to be able to reduce and prevent cardiovascular disease, as well as certain types of cancers, high blood pressure, lower blood sugar levels and reduces elevated cholesterol all of which are associated with type 2 diabetes. Magnesium's lack of absorption can be contributed to dietary fats, lactose, phosphate, phytate and oxalate. In its deficient state it is related to renal failure, which many diabetics find their self on dialysis treatment. Diabetic acidosis causes the loss of magnesium in the urine.

Food Sources:

Almonds, apples, apricots, avocados, beet tops, berries, black walnuts, brazil nuts, cabbage, cashews, coconuts, crabs, beans (soya), bread, cereals (whole grain), brewer's yeast, buckwheat (flour), dulse, figs, garlic, green peas, green vegetables, legumes, peanuts, pecans, potatoes (skin), raisins, rye, spinach, seafood, walnuts, water-cress, and yellow corn.

Inhibitors: Refine flour, bread, dairy products, fats, foods containing oxalates (rhubarb, spinach), proteins, and phytate found in wheat bran and breads.

Daily Recommended Allowance: 350 to 700 mg

Absorption: Magnesium absorbs better in the body with calcium (for every milligram of magnesium there is 2 milligrams of calcium), vitamin B-1, B-6, C, D, phosphorus, protein, zinc

Inhibitors:
The RDA is 400 mg, however, because of the deficiency diabetics need to raise their intake to 1,000 mg.

Vitamin B6 (Pyridoxine)

The nutritional deficiency of magnesium in diabetics inhibits the proper utilization of vitamin B complex, especially vitamin B6 and B12. This complexity of micronutrients is responsible for blood sugar metabolism and protects diabetics from developing neuropathy according to James F. Balch, MD and Mark Stengler, ND. [83] Vitamin B6 is also an intricate part of magnesium absorption. It inhibits glycosylation of glucose and protein formation, which eliminates the destruction of the cellular protein, decreasing the likelihood of autoimmune disease and other diabetic complications. According to Chandra Mohan, PhD the levels of B6 in diabetics is low resulting in high blood glucose levels, reducing the insulin responses and circulation.[84] She explains how over time the low level of B6 and high glucose level increase the risk of eye, kidneys, nervous, and vascular system damage.

Dr Alan Gaby, MD, reported how B6 deficient patients were also deficient in Tryptophan[x], which leads to an excessive production of Xanthurenic acid[xi] (XA). A study conducted by Charles L. Jones, D.P.M and Virgilio Gonzalez, MD of 10 type 1 diabetics with peripheral neuropathy found these patients to excrete more XA then diabetics without neuropathy. After administering 50 mg of B6 three times a day for 6 weeks the XA execration became normal and the neuropathy symptoms disappeared in all 10 patients, which suggest the B6 deficiency had been corrected.[85]

---

[x] Tryptophan is an essential neurotransmitter amino acid that works primarily in the central nervous system controlling sleep, depression, anxiety, pain

[xi] Xanthurenic acid: is a by product of Tryptophan metabolism.

B_6 (Pyridoxine) vitamin is a member of the B complex family that is widely used within the body affecting the physical and mental heath of a person and is essential for hormone production, protein digestion and absorption, as well as brain function. Pyridoxine is vital in the balance of sodium and potassium, which reduces the elevation of blood pressure and is involved in fat metabolism to decrease the prevalence of atherosclerosis, which all are closely associated with type 2 diabetes. It works to assist in the reversal of neuropathy that many diabetics are plagued with. Pyridoxine has the ability to reduce cholesterol and prevalence of heart attack and/or stroke by inhibiting the toxic chemical homocysteine and it can be useful in leg ulcer that won't heal. The destruction of B6 (Pyridoxine) is through food processing and over cooking foods.

Recommended Daily Allowance (RDA): Children-2 mgs   Adults-2 mgs   Pregnant woman-2.5 mgs

Food Sources:

Asparagus, bananas, beans (red kidney), beef, blackstrap molasses, brewers yeast, broccoli, Brussels sprouts, cabbage, cantaloupe, carrots, cauliflower, eggs, hearts, kidneys, lentils, liver, milk, onions, peanuts, pecans, green peppers, nuts, seeds, squash, vegetables green leafy, wheat bran, and wheat germ.

Absorbents:
B complex, vitamin C, magnesium, zinc, and linoleic acid. It provides the catalyst for the absorption of vitamin B 12 and protein synthesizing.

Inhibitors: Vitamin B6 is inhibited by alcohol, high protein consumption, oral contraceptive, processed foods.

Vitamin B12 (Cyanocobalmin)

In his book *How to Prevent and Treat Diabetes with Natural Medicine*, Michael T. Murray, ND discusses the fact that Vitamin B12 has been successful in treating diabetic neuropathy; however, it is unclear whether the success is due to correcting B12 deficiency or normalizing B12 metabolic balance in diabetics. Dr. Murray states "diabetic neuropathy is very similar to that of classical B12 deficiency. A typical symptom of B12 deficiency is megaloblastic anemia which is characterized by abnormal red blood cells in the bone marrow." [86] Vitamin B12 is another important element in the stabilization of diabetes not only to prevent neuropathy, but also in the absorption of vitamin B5, which assist in reducing hypoglycemia and balances Cortisones, other adrenal hormones and reduce painful burning feet that sometimes affect diabetics.[87]

In order for the proper digestion, absorption and assimilation of proteins, carbohydrates and fats Cyanocobalmin is required. As we have seen when food is unable to digest, absorb or assimilate in the body there is weight gain or obesity, which could lead to diabetes. When Cyanocobalmin teams up with folic acid they inhibit the formation of the amino acid Homocysteine. Homocysteine is responsible for the elevation of cholesterol, heart disease, and stroke that are sometimes seen in diabetics. I have successful used this combination along with specific herbs to assist my clients in reducing their blood pressure and diabetes. Cyanocobalmin is administered in a sublingual form in order to be absorbed in the blood stream and not have to go through the digestive tract.

Cyanocobalmin is either intravenously, sublingual, or time released capsule administered because of the intrinsic factor with the stomach. The intrinsic factor of the stomach assists in protecting Cyanocobalmin (B12) from stomach acid so it can be absorbed in the first part of the small intestine. The intrinsic factor is low in most humans reducing its ability to assist Cyanocobalmin move safely through the stomach. When B12 is in a multivitamin, the other vitamins help to protect it allowing it to move through the stomach into the intestines Cyanocobalmin is best absorbed when combined with vitamin B complex, B3, Vitamin C, calcium, choline, folic acid, inositol, potassium, and sodium.

Daily Recommended Allowance: Children .7 mcg 2-3 mcg Adults 2.0 mcg

Absorption Contributors: Vitamin B 12 absorbs best when combined with Calcium, Choline, Folic Acid, Inositol, Potassium, Sodium, Vitamin B complex, B6, vitamin C,

Inhibiters: gastrointestinal disorders, alcohol, low hydrochloric stomach acid, tobacco smoking.

Food Sources:

Alfalfa (herb), bananas, bee pollen, bladder wrack (seaweed), brewers yeast, comfrey leaves (herb), cottage cheese, cheese, chicken, concord dulse (seaweed), grapes, desiccated liver, eggs, herring, hops (herb), kelp (seaweed), kombu (seaweed), (meat) kidney, lamb, mackerel, milk, nori (seaweed), oysters, peanuts, sardines, shrimp, sunflower seeds, tuna, turkey, and wheat germ,

Vitamin C (Ascorbic Acid)

Researchers from the Centers for Disease Control and Prevention characterized the importance of vitamin C in a diabetic study of 237 newly diagnosed diabetic patients and 1,803 non-diabetic patients. They found lower blood serum levels of vitamin C in diabetic patients than in non-diabetics. They concluded that future research should measure and account for the influence of vitamin C as a major factor in diabetes.[88] Even in their research they considered other factors as a cause of reduced vitamin C, however, they did not consider the fact that Vitamin C degrades in an acid environment and need the full range of B vitamins to be absorbed. Nor for that matter did they link the relationship between vitamin C and magnesium, which are all present factors of diabetes. They did on the other hand consider dietary habits, tobacco use and the health status of the participants in the study.

Studies show diabetic have cellular vitamin C deficiencies, because the proper balance of insulin is needed to enhance its absorption, however, without the balance of vitamin C diabetics encounter a host of other conditions including poor wound healing, an increase in the tendency to bleed, and an elevation in their cholesterol levels leading to cardiovascular disease, vascular disease, and impaired immune system.[89] "Vitamin C supplementation has shown to exert a mild effect in improving glucose control, as evident by a slightly lower A_1C in the vitamin C group 8.5 percent compared to a placebo 9.3 percent in one double blind study," comments Michael Murray, ND. He went on to say, "Probably more important than any significant effect on improving blood sugar control is the fact that vitamin C supplementation has been shown to reduce the formation of compounds linked to the development of diabetic complications such as Sorbitol.[xii] [90] When the body's vitamin C levels are balanced through supplementation it maintains a healthy blood glucose level. In a 12 month study at the University of Australia where 500 mg of vitamin C was administrated to 20 diabetics, they found after 9 months the diabetic vitamin C levels improved and their albumin[xiii] excretion rate reduced over the placebo group. The University of Vienna study conducted by Professor R. Pfleger and colleagues, which was published in a European journal of internal medicine in 1937 shows 300 to 500 mg/day of vitamin C, reduced high glucose blood levels by 30% and lowered daily insulin requirements by 27%. The study also showed supplementation of vitamin C eliminated sugar in the urine of diabetics.[91]

Vitamin C has amazing benefits to the body. It has been shown that many diabetics have elevated cholesterol and high blood pressure, which vitamin C reduces both and improves the good cholesterol as it assists in preventing atherosclerosis. It's a powerful wound healer in large doses, having the ability to assist diabetics in healing wounds thus preventing amputation of limbs. Vitamin C assists in the metabolism of amino acids (protein), especially the neurotransmitter hormones epinephrine and norepinephrine. It also promotes the synthesizing of hormones from the adrenals. Vitamin C together in combination with vitamin E is powerful antioxidants and can be used by diabetic to reduce free radical that can cause cancer. In the body vitamin C works to assist food in being absorbed and transferred into energy.

Good Food Sources:

Asparagus, avocados, beet (greens), black currants, broccoli, Brussels sprouts, cabbage, cantaloupe, cauliflower, chard (Swiss),

---

[xii] Sorbitol is a sugar molecule produced by the body formed from glucose conversion within the cell. An increase of Sorbitol in the cell can cause it to leak vital nutrients such as amino acids, inositol, glutathione, niacin, magnesium, potassium and vitamin C, which damages the cell. Murray Michael, ND, How to Prevent and Treat Diabetes with Natural Medicine.

[xiii] Albumin is a protein in blood plasma that maintains the integrity of the blood vessels, tissues and assists the blood in circulating hormones, and certain drugs. The Merck Manual of Medical Information

collards, dandelion (greens), dulse, grapefruit, green peppers, kale, kiwi fruit, lemons, limes, mangos, melons, mustard (greens), onions, oranges, papayas, peas, sweet peppers, persimmons, pineapple, radishes, rose hips (herb), spinach, strawberries, tomatoes, turnip (greens), and watercress.

RDA: Children 300-500 mg Adults 600-1,000 mg   smokers 2,000-3,000 mg

Note: however it is noted that vitamin C can be taken from 800 to 10,000 a day. There is no toxicity with this vitamin, however when the body becomes overloaded the bowels become loose. I recommend 3,000 to 5,000 mg a day to my clients and have them administer vitamin C in 1,000 inclement throughout the day. But dividing the dosage it reduces the loose stools and is able to absorb in the body. The literature states the maximum dose taken in one seating is 3,000 mg and anything over that in the same seating in not absorbed.

Absorption Contributors: Vitamin C is easier absorbed with bioflavonoid, calcium, magnesium, multi minerals potassium, sodium, zinc, and vitamin D.

Inhibitors: Alcohol, fried food, oral contraceptives, steroids and tobacco smoking.

Vitamin E

Researchers from the University Hospital, Queen's Medical Centre, Nottingham, England, found that 70% of the diabetic patients died from fatty deposits lodged in their arteries and two-to four-fold excess mortality in those with impaired glucose tolerance.[92]

Reduced blood levels of vitamin E, contributes to the risk of type 2 diabetes according to Dr. Robert C. Atkins, founder of the Atkins Clinic in New York City. He stated, that "Blood platelets in diabetics contain less vitamin E than platelets of non-diabetics. When vitamin E levels are low, the risk of acquiring Type 2 diabetes rises by a ratio of nearly four to one." He continued by citing a study where 100 International Units (IU) a day of vitamin E was administered for 3 months to type 1 diabetics. The conclusion of the study showed a significant reduction in high blood sugar tissue damage, as well as the decrease in triglycerides and heart disease risk.[93] Vitamin E has not only shown to address diabetic complications, it also protects the body from free radical damage, glycosylation and cardiovascular disease. Type 2-diabetes is a major risk factor of cardiovascular disease. The Cambridge Heart Antioxidant Study (CHAOS) double blind placebo research of 2,002 patients receiving 400-800 IUs of vitamin E supplements for 510 days showed 75 percent fewer heart attacks then the placebo group.[94] In a short 3-month study of 25 elderly diabetics who received 900 IU of vitamin E daily showed a significant decrease in their A1C levels (blood sugar levels), triglycerides, cholesterol (HDL and LDL), and their risk of ischemic heart disease.[95]

Vitamin E will assist in wound healing of a diabetic and prevent atherosclerosis from developing. As an antioxidant it promotes circulation for tissue growth as it prevents cardiovascular disease and act as an antioxidant. Also vitamin E has been known to reduce elevated blood pressure. Vitamin E intake is known to improve the uptake of insulin, decreasing elevated blood sugar levels. In the body vitamin E prevents the oxidation of other fatty acids (vitamin A, D, and essential fatty acids).

RDA: 300 international units (IU) daily

Note: Vitamin E can safely be taken up to 1,200 IU.

Absorption Contributors:
This vitamin is more effectively absorbed when accompanied by Inositol, Manganese and selenium, Vitamin A, B Complex, C, F.

Good Food Sources:

Broccoli, brown rice, Brussels Sprouts, cereal (whole grain), dulse, eggs, kelp, leafy green vegetables, liver (desiccated), milk, oatmeal, oil (vegetable), meat (organ), peas, peanuts, potatoes (sweet), salmon, sardines, sesame seeds, soybeans, spinach, sunflower seeds, tuna, watercress, wheat, and wheat germ.

Selenium

Selenium is another nutrient that assists in the stimulation of glucose uptake, glycosis[xiv], gluconeogenesis[xv] and fatty acid synthesis. It was found in a Vienna, Austria research study of 20 type 1 diabetics and 20 non-diabetics that the selenium red blood cell levels were lower then the non-diabetics. The study also showed when there are low levels of selenium in diabetic patients; it contributes to low levels of glutathione peroxide activity resulting in unnecessary bleeding. [96] However, in most studies selenium is a risk factor for type 2 diabetes.

Selenium has shown promise in its ability to reduce elevated cholesterol and lower high blood pressure as well as assisting the pancreas in its metabolic function. As a powerful antioxidant it protects against cancer causing free radicals and protects the heart.

RDA: Children 100-300 mcg Woman 450-750 mcg   Men 400-700 mcg Women who are pregnant should not take over 40 mcg a day.

Absorption Contributors:
In order for Selenium absorption vitamin A, E is needed.

Good food sources include:

Alfalfa, brewer's yeast, broccoli, brown rice, burdock root, cabbage, chicken, cod, cottage cheese, dulse (seaweed), eggs, garlic, herring, kelp, molasses, mushrooms, nuts (Brazil), onions, oysters, parsley, salmon, tuna, vegetables (most all), wheat germ, whole grains, zucchini.

Inhibitors: High volumes of Vitamin C, Heavy metals (cadmium, lead, mercury, etc), chemotherapy drugs, zinc and other trace minerals.

Selenium should not be taken with vitamin C because they will inhibit each other. Refined foods and treated and processed foods also inhibit Selenium.

[xiv]   Glucosis is enzymatic breakdown of carbohydrate.
[xv]   Gluconeogenesis is the transformation of fats and proteins into glucose.

Niacin

Niacin vitamin B3 is an essential asset in glucose tolerance factor, making it an important element in preventing, reducing and/or eliminating diabetes and hypoglycemia. In its form as niacin amide, vitamin B3 has been researched as a possible element to prevent new cases of type 1-diabetes. Trail studies have shown in larger dosages it assists in restoring beta-cells or slowing down their destruction.[97] Not only is niacin major in diabetes, but also it is also essential in reducing the LDL levels that cause complications (cardiovascular, obesity, etc.) of type 1 and 2 diabetes.[98] Because of it flushing nature niacin by it self is hard on a diabetic's system, so they should take niacin in the form of inosital hexaniacinate for best result (inositol is an unofficial member of the B vitamin complex). Time released niacin is toxic to the liver and should be the last resort.

It was show in a study of 153 patients treated with 600-1,800 mg of inositol hexaniacinate three times per day reduced their cholesterol levels by eighteen percent with a 16% decrease in triglycerides as their HDL's increased thirty percent.[99]

Niacin (B3) is a member of the B vitamin family that aids in the metabolic process of digesting, absorbing, and assimilating nutrients from food in the body. Part of its role is to balance blood sugar levels as well as decrease elevated cholesterol levels in the blood. Niacin aids the body in reducing stress lowering the prevalence of high blood pressure. It also improves body circulation that assist diabetics and reduces the incidents of limb wounds and amputations.

RDA: Children 50-130 mg   Woman 130-150 mg   Men 150-200 mg

Note: The younger a man or woman is the more of this vitamin they will take.

Absorption Contributors

Niacin is best absorbed when taken in conjunction with vitamin B complex, B1, B2, Vitamin C, and chromium.

Good Food Sources:

Alfalfa, asparagus, brewer's yeast, broccoli, burdock root, cabbage, carrots, cauliflower, cheese, chicken, flour (corn), dates, eggs, fish (mackerel), greens (dandelion), milk, mushrooms, peanuts, potatoes, salmon, squash, tomatoes, tuna, turkey, wheat germ, whole wheat products, zucchini.

Inhibitors: Alcohol, antibiotics, coffee, oral contraception, tobacco smoking,

Note: Niacin causes the body to flush with a tingling sensation over the body. The better forms of niacin are the non-flush type or niacinamide, which do not cause the flushing sensation.

Biotin

Studies indicate that diabetics have a very low level of biotin a member of the B vitamin family. Biotin deficiency impairs the sensitivity of sugar metabolism by the liver because of its ability to increase the enzyme glucokinase, which is responsible for the synthesizing of sugar by the liver. Biotin has shown to improve blood glucose levels and reduce fasting blood sugar levels in type 1 diabetics when given 16 mg a day.[100] In a study appearing on Renal Failure, 11 regular (1-7 years) hemodialysis diabetic patients ages ranging 32-76 received high doses of biotin intervene as part of an oral glucose tolerance test. At the conclusion of the study it was found that 75% of the participant glucose levels reduced substantially. The authors of the study concluded by stating "Our results offers support to the findings of other studies about the beneficial effects of biotin in experimental or clinical diabetes mellitus, and argue for the involvement of biotin in glucose metabolism."[101] Blood glucose levels significantly improve in one study where 16 milligrams a day of biotin was administered to type 1 diabetic and 9 milligrams to type 2 diabetics. Biotin has also improved diabetic neuropathy (nerve damage).[102]

The importance of Biotin in the case of diabetics is its ability to assist the body in using essential fats. These are fatty aid the body uses to balance blood sugar levels and reduce excess fat. It also assists in the digestive process of carbohydrates, fats, and proteins. Biotin promotes the absorption of vitamin B complex and stimulates the growth of nervous tissues. It aids the absorption of ascorbic acid (vitamin C), B complex, magnesium, and manganese.

RDA: Children 100-150mcg   Adults 300-1,000mcg

Absorption Contributors: vitamin B complex, B12, Folic acid, Pantothenic Acid, vitamin C, Sulfur and healthy gut flora.

Signs of Deficiencies: dermatitis, depression, eczema, dandruff, skin disorders, loss of appetite, Anemia, nausea, alopecia, hallucinations, muscle pain, drowsiness, baldness,

Causes of Deficiencies: Raw egg whites (because it contains an element known as avidin, which inhibits Biotins absorption.) and fried foods chronic alcohol drinking, antibiotics, and cradle cap. There have not been any reports of toxicity in high dosage of this vitamin.

Sources: Almond, Barley, Beef liver, Black-eyed peas, Bran, Brewer's yeast, Brown rice, Cauliflower, Cereal (whole wheat), Cranberries, Egg yolk, Lentils, Liver (Beef, Lamb), Mushrooms, Oatmeal, Peanut butter, Peanut roasted, Pecans, Rice bran, Rice germ, Polished Rice, Salmon, Sardines (canned), Soy (beans, flour), Split peas, Textured vegetable protein (TVP), and Walnuts.

Inhibitors: Alcohol, antibiotics

Inositol

Inositol is not officially a B vitamin, but many researchers classify it in that category. One of the reasons diabetics are deficient in inositol is because they excrete large amount of it in their urine, resulting in neuropathy, according to Robert Matz, M.D. Dr. Matz stated "Reduced magnesium in diabetic patients can reduce inositol transport by 50%. He continued by saying "Inositol and myoinositol deficiency can be important factors in some of the underlying complications of chronic diabetes."[103] Inositol is important to type 2 diabetics because when teamed up with Choline they form lecithin a phospholipids that lowers cholesterol and nourishes the brain. It is noted by Adelle Davis that when recovering heart attack patients receive 2,000 mg Choline and 750 mg inositol their cholesterol levels drastically decrease. [104]

As a member of the lipotropic family, Inositol prevents fat build up in the liver and has the ability to protect and reverse degeneration of the myelin sheathing of the nervous system, which is essential in many diabetics who have neuropathy. The deficiency of either Inositol or Choline inhibits the production of lecithin. Lecithin is a cholesterol lowering substance that also nourishes brain cells (I will elaborate on lecithin later). Inositol reduces the prevalence of arteriosclerosis.

RDA: none established: However, it has been suggested that it can be consumed from 12 grams for depression, to between 100-500 mg for liver disorders and between 1,000-2,000 for diabetes.

Requirement for Absorption: Vitamin B Complex, B12, Choline, Linoleic acid, and iron magnesium. There have not been any known toxic affects from this vitamin.

Signs of Deficiencies: Baldness, depression, diabetes, constipation, eczema, elevated cholesterol, eye disorders, liver disorders, liver disorders, Multiple Sclerosis,

Inhibitors: Alcohol, antibiotics, birth control pills, caffeine in large amounts, diuretics, phytates.

Good Food Sources:

Beans (cooked), Beans (green), Brewers yeast, Cantaloupe, Citrus fruit, Corn, Eggs, Fish, Lecithin, Legumes, Meats, Molasses (unrefined), Nuts, Oatmeal (unprocessed), Raisins, Soy flour, Vegetables, and Whole wheat bread (stone ground).

Vanadium

There are not many elements that actually mimic insulin and last for weeks after it has been administered like vanadium. Animal studies have shown vanadium has the ability to lower glucose levels and its effect can last for ten weeks. In a 1996 study where 50 milligram of vanadyl sulfate was administered twice a day to eight men and women with type 2 diabetes for four weeks; this group of participants where also given a placebo for an additional four weeks. The result of the study was showed their fasting glucose levels decreased by 20 percent well into the placebo period.[105]

Vanadium stimulates GLUT-4 transporters[xvi] carry glucose inside the cell in the same manner as insulin. Julian Whitaker, MD, says, "Vanadium has been identified as one of the few compounds other than insulin that can activate GLUT-4 transporters.[106] There is a rumor of vanadium's toxicity however, according to John McNeil, a world expert on vanadium, Dean of the Faculty of Pharmaceutical Sciences at the University of British Columbia, states it is just a rumor based on only one research study with no other studies to maintain the theory. High doses of 400 mg of vanadium have been safely consumed with only reports of diarrhea. Diabetic have been given 150 mg a day with success. [107] It was noted by Barbara F. Harland, PhD., R.D. and B.A. Harden-Williams M.S. of Howard University in Washington, D.C. that "Pharmacologic doses of the mineral 10 to 100 times the normal intake can alter cholesterol and triglyceride metabolism, as well as the shape of red blood cells and stimulate glucose oxidation and glycogen synthesis in the liver."[108] Because of Vanadium's ability to lower glucose levels, it also lowers blood pressure according to the University of British Columbia, Vancouver, Canada.[109] With an understanding of vanadium's ability to not only lower glucose levels, but also reduce blood pressure (It has the ability to balance sodium and potassium), triglycerides, and cholesterol we can see the benefits of its use with type 2 diabetics, because many of them have hypertension, elevated cholesterol, and are overweight. This is not to say that type 1 diabetics will not benefit from vanadium.

Vanadium aids in the reduction of cholesterol and improves the utilization of insulin. It decreases the prevalence of cardiovascular disease, which some diabetics suffer from. However, it is a hard mineral for the body to absorb.

RDA: 100 to 600 mg
Sources of Absorption:

Inhibitors: There are no known interactions with food or other elements.

[xvi] GLUT-4 transporters signaling protein resides within the cell to raise the cell's membrane, in order for them to grab onto glucose and take deliver it inside the cell.

Good Food Sources:

Black pepper, soy oil, corn oil, olive oil, and olives

Zinc

Zinc is an essential mineral forming the DNA and RNA, as well as being a component of most body tissues, influencing hormones and all glandular processes. Zinc is the co-factor in several hundred enzymatic processes and is involved in virtually all aspects of insulin metabolism including synthesis, secretion, and utilization of insulin. Zinc is known to protect beta cells from destruction and has an antiviral effect promoting wound healing, which assist diabetics in healing leg ulcers. Zinc deficiencies have been found in type 1 and type 2 diabetics, because of the excessive amount of zinc excreted in their urine. [110]

In the Tennessee based Surgical Research Laboratories study of 37 obese patients they found high levels of zinc concentrated in their urine, contributing to low blood levels of zinc. The finding of the study was to measure copper and zinc levels in obese patients, which showed deficient zinc blood levels and notably above normal copper levels determining that obese patients who are at high risk of diabetes have a zinc and cooper deficiencies. This study indicated that the majority of type 2 diabetics have deficiencies of both zinc and copper, although there are some reports that conflict with zinc's ability to prevent diabetes. [111]

Zinc has the ability to normalize insulin and balance the blood sugar levels because it is a component of insulin. It is a powerful wound healer, immune stimulator and is an essential mineral found in all cells because it aids in the formulation of RNA and DNA. Zinc reduces cholesterol levels in the blood and is a major mineral in the function of the reproductive system, especially the prostate. It is also known for it antioxidant properties and is essential in the function of the nervous system.

RDA: 15 to 30 mg

Absorption Contributing Substances:

To absorb in the body this mineral needs vitamin A, vitamin B6, calcium, copper, hydrochloric acid, magnesium, phosphorus.

Inhibiting Substances:

Alcohol, calcium (high amounts), copper (high amounts), protein (low intake), rhubarb, spinach, sugar (excessive amounts), stress, wheat.

Good food sources:

Brewers Yeast, Brazil nuts, cashews, chicken, dulse, eggs (yolk), fish (herring, tuna), kelp, legumes, lecithin (soy), lima beans, meats (liver), mushrooms, oysters, peanuts, pecans, pumpkin, sardines, seafood, seeds, soybeans, sunflower seeds, and whole grains.

Vitamin D (Cholecalciferol) = D3; Ergocalciferol = D2

Vitamin D is an important element in insulin secretion and the glucose tolerance factor. When deficient it causes other type 2 diabetic complication including cataracts and cardiovascular disease. An interview with B.J. Boucher, M.D., of the Royal London School of Medicine and Dentistry in England Published in Clinical Pearls, health journal stated, "Vitamin D is needed by the islet cells to secrete insulin normally. This may happen since it helps to ensure an adequate supply of calcium, upon which many enzymes related to insulin secretions and releases are dependent." He continued, "vitamin D can improve insulin resistance with a reduction in hyper-insulinemia (high levels of insulin in the blood), along with an improvement in glucose tolerance when given in early stages of glucose intolerance in kidney disease. The latter develops when vitamin D is not properly formed."[112]

Vitamin D is found in human skin tissues and is acquired from sun-light. When it enters the skin and penetrates the blood it is transformed by a cholesterol component to vitamin D3. It helps in the prevention skin disease from Ultraviolet light and other air borne pollutants. The primary function of vitamin D includes calcium and phosphorus intestinal absorption and their ability to be deposited in the bones. It also has a major part in the extraction of calcium and phosphorus from the bones. Vitamin D is a fat-soluble vitamin, playing two roles, one as a vitamin and the other as a hormone. As part of it job vitamin D regulates heart rhythms and can prevent the prevalence of celiac disease, which is a disease the many diabetics come down with especially type 1 diabetic.

RDA: Children 300-400 IU   Woman 400 IU   Men 400 IU

Absorption Contributors:

Calcium and Phosphorus, vitamin A, Choline, C, F.

Inhibitors:

Lack of sun-light, fried foods, liver and kidney disease (dialysis and kidney stones).

Good sources of vitamin D:

Cod liver oil, cottage cheese, dairy products, dandelion greens, eggs yolks, halibut, herring, mackerel, oatmeal, oysters, salmon, sardines, sweet potatoes, tuna, and vegetable oil.

Exercise

"One of the benefits of physical activity is to dilate (expand) the network of blood vessels so blood reaches the muscles and vital organs as well as the small capillaries. When a person does not exercise, this expansion of the circulatory system is diminished."

Susan M. Lark, M.D., James A. Richards, M.B.A.
The Chemistry of Success

Major factors of type 2 diabetes are the lack of physical activity, high fat intake, refined carbohydrates, processed foods, and junk foods, which increases weight gain resulting in diabetes. A National Institute of Health (NIH) in Bethesda, Maryland survey indicated that a low fat eating habit and walking for a half hour a day or other exercises would reduce the risk of developing diabetes by 58% amongst high risk groups. In NIH's 3 year study of 3,234 overweight and hyperglycemic volunteers, they found the individuals who were introduced to health lifestyle changes lost an average of 15 pounds. [113]

Exercise has not only shown to improve blood sugar levels of type 2 diabetic, but the study at the Ohio State University College of Medicine at Columbia indicated that exercise increases insulin sensitivity and reduces high blood glucose levels.[114]

Exercise can be of any type, I recommend Tai Chi, Yoga, Qi Gong because not only are they cardiovascular exercises, but they work on the internal body (organs) as well. They have specific posture for different organs. These exercises provide the organs with the stimuli that is needed to assist in it ability to function at its optimum. The postures will create a balance with in the organs that will assist it in moving into its healing process. The postures work well with a good choice of foods and supplementation to decrease the elevated glucose levels and any other complications.

The slow consistent movement of Tai Chi and Qi Gong not only improves circulation of the blood but also reduces blood sugar levels, overweight conditions, high blood pressure, and elevated cholesterol. Both of the exercises synchronize the breath with the movements. A major part of Qi Gong is the coordination of movement and breath, which promotes oxygenation of the blood. Oxygenation of the blood improves its circulation as well as balances the relationship between cells, glucose and insulin promoting a positive acceptance of glucose lowers the amount of glucose in the blood. These exercises reduce stress levels again, promoting the free flow of blood reducing the high glucose levels and working on decreasing weight, this is a major part of type 2 diabetes. Because they create circulation Tai Chi and Qi Gong, improve the nervous system function reducing neuropathy and limb amputations.

Research from the Beijing University of Chinese Medicine and Pharmacology found that after consistently performing Qi Gong exercises diabetic patients blood sugar levels decrease and 42.9% of them reduced their medication for their diabetes.

On the other hand, research has come out showing the value of yoga in the reduction and/or eliminating of high blood glucose levels. In an article published in the Indian Journal of Physiology and Pharmacology, entitled "Effect of Yoga asana on nerve condition in type 2 diabetes". The study showed where middle aged participants with type 2 diabetes where guided consistently through yoga asana (postures) for 40 days and at the end of that period there was a significant decrease in their fasting blood glucose levels. The levels decreased between 61.7 mg/dl to 100 mg/dl. The conclusion of this study suggests that when yoga is used with type 2 diabetics there is a greater glucose control and pulmonary function. [115]

The two studies indicate that these Chinese and Ayurvedic forms of exercise have a great effect on the balancing and lowering elevated glucose levels in a matter of days when preformed on a consistent regular basis. Also exercises that incorporate the mind, body and spirit to create a relaxing balanced feeling that assist the body in balancing glucose levels.

Complications of Diabetes

"It is far easier and safer to prevent illness by curing illness which has been brought on by our own ignorance and carelessness. Hence, it is the duty of all thoughtful men to understand the law of health."

Gandhi Health Guide

Over the years of a diabetic's life their body and the disease increase their risk for other type of health conditions such as cardiovascular disease, which causes 65 percent of diabetic's deaths.[116] Much of the Cardiovascular Disease (CVD) found with diabetics is related to atherosclerosis a disease that affects the arterial blood supply to the heart, not only dose it cause CVD, but also contributes to stroke and high blood pressure. Atherosclerosis, is harden of the inner and middle walls of the arteries reducing it's elasticity resulting in a thicker wall restricting blood flow to the organs and brain. Coronary Artery Disease can be caused by atherosclerosis where fat deposits and cholesterol build up along the walls of the arteries creating narrowing restricting and blocking blood flow to the heart decreasing the hearts function and causing it to work harder. Over a period of time calcium deposits can accumulate in an atheroma[xvii] resulting in a blood clot (thrombus)[xviii]

[xvii] A deposit or degenerative accumulation of lipid-containing plaques on the innermost layer of the wall of an artery. American Heritage Dictionary

[xviii] A fibrinous clot formed in a blood vessel or in a chamber of the heart. American Heritage Dictionary

blocking more of the artery; if the blood clot detaches (embolus)[xix] and float through the blood vessels it can reach the brain resulting in stroke or death. CVD has a direct link to ones eating habits and the amount of fat and sugar (sugar also turns to fat) consumed.

Homocysteine a Danger to Life

Homocysteine, caused by a nutritional deficiency of folic acid, vitamin B6, and B12,[117] is responsible for contributing to atherosclerosis where it damages the walls of the arteries, interrupting collagen production and according to the American Journal of Cardiology restrict blood flow. [118]

The amino acid methionine is the body's natural creator of Homocysteine. Homocysteine occurs during the conversion of methionine to cysteine. Homocysteine is only damaging to the body when it is in excessive levels. Methionine in excessive levels causes a vitamin B_6, vitamin B_{12}, and folic acid deficiency resulting in dangerous high levels of homocysteine.[119] Consuming large amounts of dairy products, meat products, and an increasing amount of refined sugar with a low intake of fruits and vegetables elevates homocysteine levels. The amino acid Methionine is found in low levels in the body and plays a very special role as a sulfur element aiding the formation of deoxyribonucleic acid (DNA) and ribonucleic acid (RNA).

Frank Murray in his book *Natural Supplements for Diabetes* cites a 12-week study by Robert Clarke, M.D., and associates at Radcliffe infirmary in Oxford, England, in which they administered folic acid, vitamin B_6 and vitamin B_{12} to 1,114 people to affect their blood homocysteine level. The findings were that the administration of 0.5 to 5 mg/day of folic acid, 0.5mg/day vitamin B_{12} reduced homocysteine levels by one-quarter. Clarke went on to show where foods high in folic acid lowered homocysteine levels by 25%. [120]

[xix] A mass, such as an air bubble, a detached blood clot, or a foreign body, that travels through the bloodstream and lodges so as to obstruct or occlude a blood vessel. American Heritage Dictionary.

High Blood Pressure/Hypertension

It is common to find diabetics that are overweight with elevated blood pressure. The triplet diabetes, hypertension and being overweight are referred to as Syndrome X. A large percentage of type 2 diabetics are overweight and many of them have hypertension. Normal blood pressure is 120/80. If the pressure elevates over 135/90 or higher there is a risk of cardiovascular disease and/or stroke. The elevation of the blood pressure also affects diabetic's eyes, kidneys and nervous system. Oxidative stress, improper eating habits, high levels of homocysteine, overweight, and obesity age, high cholesterol, and lack of exercise are major causes for the blood pressure to elevate.

When a person's sodium intake is too high relative to their potassium intake, they disrupt the delicate chemical balance of the cells resulting in elevated blood pressure. This is why in many cases of hypertension the physician prescribes medication with potassium (diuretic) and recommends that their patients reduce or eliminate their sodium intake. Another reason for hypertension is atherosclerosis where the blood vessels become hard and restrictive and the blood is unable to flow properly (this topic has already been discussed above).

Smoking contributes to high blood pressure and diabetes. There are over 4,000 different harmful chemicals in tobacco, made up of many different type substances including heavy metals, battery acid, formaldehyde and more. One of the major ingredients in tobacco is the heavy metal cadmium, known to elevate the blood pressure. In many instances when the blood pressure becomes so high that a person has to continually switch medications to control their blood pressure, than the cause could be from heavy metal like cadmium and/or lead poisoning[121] causing nutritional deficiencies of low levels of zinc in women or higher copper values.[122] Cigarette smoking also increases cholesterol and other factor of increased blood pressure. High blood pressure is a contributing factor in stroke.

Overweight/Obesity

"The body is like a very finely tuned engine. The wrong fuel, delivered at the wrong rate, with other fuels or contaminants mixed in, will generally immediately impair the engine's performance and eventually just shut down the engine."

Thomas E. Levy, M.D., J.D.
Optimal Nutrition for Optimal Health

Being overweight, up to the point of obesity, is the leading risk factor for type 2 diabetes, coronary heart disease, high blood pressure, elevated cholesterol, stroke, gallbladder disease, osteoarthritis, cancer, etc. According to the National Health and Nutrition Examination Survey (NHANES) 2001 to 2004 two-thirds of the adults living in the United States are overweight or obese.[123] The survey also pointed out that 16% of children 9 through 19 are also overweight or obese. Obesity has become a pandemic in the United States.[124]

When your body weight exceeds the standard set for your desirable weight, but is not excessively above the standard, it is categorized as overweight. A person is obese when they have an excessive, abnormal amount of body fat. This amount exceeds all weight standards. It is true that a person can be overweight and not obese; however, both conditions are risk factors for several types of diseases.

Body weight is calculated by a system known as the Body Mass Index (BMI). The BMI is a system to calculate weight by height to determine where your weight is in reference to the standards of underweight, normal weight, overweight or obese. Following this is the BMI chart and instructions how to use the chart in order to calculate your body mass index.

The cause of overweight and obesity is malabsorption of nutrients that leads to malnutrition of the cells allowing waste by product from the foods to accumulate in the small intestine and leak into the blood stream where it aligns itself with adipose tissue (fatty tissues). The merge of the two create a growth and expansion into the tissue where they spread throughout the body putting pressures on organs, bones, and systems. The expansion of the waste and adipose tissue inhibits organ, bones and systems function to the point where they malfunction increasing the risk of many types of diseases.

Medical science views this pandemic as one of heredity and lifestyle. Looking at it from a different view we may possibly say that both of these could be the cause, however, a key element in this pandemic is our food supply and the understanding of how to eat to live and not live to eat. The latter is what we have been trained to do. Eating like many other things is a learned behavior. Many times when we learn something it becomes part of our daily life and heard to change and eating is one of those things.

When foods are eaten in any type of combination it confuses the body and the body does not know which enzymes to use in order to digest the food partials. Results of this is food accumulating in the small intestine for an extended period of time, causing distention of the abdomen and the possibility of waste leaking in the blood stream consequentialy increasing the risk of elevated cholesterol, hypertension, diabetes, heart disease and other health issues.

The other issue with overweight and obesity is the lack of exercise. Our society consumes a lot of refined foods with empty calories, junk foods, fried, sugary foods with no nutritional values. Many of us don't take the time to burn these calories off so they lodge their self in the adipose tissue of the body and continue to accumulate. Bad eating habits are affecting our children at a rapid rate, especially in this age of video games and the educational system taking physical education out of the schools.

According to the Center for Disease Control and Prevention childhood obesity has doubled over the past 20 years for children ages 6-11, from 6.5% in 1980 to 17.0% in 2006. The obese rate for children ages 12-19 as tripled during that time form 5% to 17.6%. Many of these children will grow into overweight or obese adults with risk of type 2 diabetes, stroke, some type of cancer or osteoarthritis. At their present age they are at risk of high blood pressure, elevated cholesterol, and cardiovascular disease.[125]

As these children grow into adults and have children of their own, their children are also at risk of overweight, obesity, type 2 diabetes, hypertension, cardiovascular dis-ease, and other health related disparities. Obesity is wider then medical science thinks it is, with its potential of reaching the next twenty or more generations if we don't put a stop to it now.

Body Mass Index

What is the Body Mass Index and How does it work and relate to diabetes?

> *Everything in this world has a hidden meaning. Men, animals, trees, stars, they are all hieroglyphics . . . When you see them, you do not understand them. You think they are really men, animals, trees, stars. It is only later that you understand.*
>
> Nikos Kazantzakis Zorba the Greek

The "Body Mass Index (BMI) is a number calculating a person's weight, height to the ratio to body fat. BMI is a reliable indicator of body fatness for people. BMI does not measure body fat directly, but research has shown that BMI correlates to direct measures of body fat, such as underwater weight and dual energy X-ray absorptiometry (DXA). BMI can be considered an alternative for direct measure of body fat. Additionally, BMI is an inexpensive and easy-to-perform method of screening for weight categories that may lead to health problems.

The BMI is a tool (not a diagnostic tool) used to screen the weight of children and adult for possible problems that could put them at risk for being overweight, or obese leading into other type of health disparities. Along with this there are other test and information needed to determine if the person is at risk of a disparity.

This is how to use the BMI chart, you would look up your height and calculate it with your height and this will provide the information needed to determine where you are in terms of being in the normal percentile, overweight or obese. Your Body Mass Index should not excess 25% of your weight. If it goes past 25 then you are in the categories of being overweight and the higher it gets the more you are moving towards obesity.

The relationship between the BMI and diabetes is one of weight gain especially in type 2. The statistic literature shows that 95 percent of the people with diabetes have type 2 and of that the mass majority are either overweight or obese. As a matter of fact, being overweight and/or obese is a very high risk factor for diabetes as well as other health disparities.

Body Mass Index Chart

The Body Mass Index chart or Quetelet index, is a statistical way of calculating a person's weight with their height to determine their health and their risk of overweight and obesity. This system dates back to the Belgian polymath Adolphe Quetelet who discovered this system between 1830 and 1850 during the course of developing "social physics."

BMI popularity came in the 1950's and 60'during the onset of the obesity alert in Western society. It is a tool for health professionals to identify the fatness or thinness of a person.

My personal opinion is that it is a great tool that needs to be readjusted for people of different cultures and backgrounds. For instance, I am 5-feet-6 inches, weighing 135 pounds. On the BMI scale I would calculate around 22. Well if 25 is overweight then that means if I gain 17 pounds I would be in the overweight category. If you have ever seen me you know that I could stand to gain 20 pounds and should not be close to being overweight.

In the chart you will find your BMI by calculating your weight with your height, which will give you your body mass index. Example: a height of 61 and a weight of 122 calculate to a BMI of 23, which is in the normal range.

Body Mass Index Chart

BMI	19	20	21	22	23	24	25	26	27	28	29	30	35	40
Height			Weight											
58	91	96	100	105	110	115	119	124	129	134	138	143	167	191
59	94	99	104	109	114	119	124	128	133	138	143	148	173	198
60	97	102	107	112	118	123	128	133	138	143	148	153	179	204
61	100	106	111	116	122	127	132	137	143	148	153	158	185	211
62	104	109	115	120	126	131	136	142	147	153	158	164	191	218
63	107	113	118	124	130	135	141	146	152	158	163	169	197	225
64	110	116	122	128	134	140	145	151	157	163	169	174	204	232
65	114	120	126	132	138	144	150	156	162	168	174	180	210	240
66	118	124	130	136	142	148	155	161	167	173	179	186	216	247
67	121	127	134	140	146	153	159	166	172	178	185	191	223	255
68	125	131	138	144	151	158	164	171	177	184	190	197	230	262
69	128	135	142	149	155	162	169	176	182	189	196	203	236	270
70	132	139	146	153	160	167	174	181	188	195	202	207	243	278
71	136	143	150	157	165	172	179	186	193	200	208	215	250	286
72	140	147	154	162	169	177	184	191	199	206	21	221	258	294
73	144	151	159	166	174	182	189	197	204	212	219	227	265	302
74	148	155	163	171	179	186	194	202	210	218	225	233	272	311
75	152	160	168	176	184	192	200	208	216	224	232	240	279	319
76	156	164	172	180	189	197	205	213	221	230	238	246	287	328

Overweight and Obesity Risk Associated With the BMI and Waist Size

BMI		Waist sizes Below or Equal to Men 40 inches Women 35 inches	Waist size Grater than Men 40 inches Women 35 inches
18.5 or less	Underweight		
18.5-24.9	Normal		
25.0-29.9	Overweight	Increased	High
30.0-34.9	Obese	High	Very High
35.0-39.9	Obese	Very High	Very High
40 or grater	Extremely Obese	Extremely High	Extremely High

Kidney Disease (Nephrotic Syndrome)

"Living in tune our constitution goes a long way in alleviating the everyday suffering and distraction we experience."

Robert Sachs
Health for Life
Secrets of Tibetan Ayurveda

Nephrotic syndrome is the accumulation of fluid in the tissues (edema) caused by the loss of protein in the urine, resulting in albumin protein levels being low in the blood. Nephritic syndrome is common in diabetics and shown in the early stages of kidney failure. Nephropathy can lead to dialysis or a kidney transplant.

When I find that a person has protein leaking in their urine I always suggest proteolytic and/or metabolic enzymes along with specific herbs to rebalance the kidney's energy and harmony. These enzymes degrade protein and have worked well for my clients. I also recommend that the person does not consume a large amount of protein because the nitrogenous waste by products of ammonia and urea place a hardship on the kidneys. The consumption of high fiber works well because the fiber absorbs some of the nitrogenous material from the blood reducing the load on the kidney. When in taking fiber, you should make sure you consume a substantial amount of liquids. You want the fiber to be well lubricated in your system.

A study of 333,544 men between thirty-five and fifty-seven with diabetes showed they where at a thirteen percent risk of nephropathy then non-diabetics and the diabetics were at greater risk of advanced kidney failure.[126] Another study indicated that the use of B6 in the early stages of nephropathy is able to prevent long-term kidney failure.[127]

Neuropathy
(Nerve Damage)

"The human being is lord and master of all the atoms contained within his body and aura. They are his subjects, the prey of his tyrannies, the beneficiaries of his wisdom and good sense."

Vera Stanley Alder
The Secret of the Atomic Age

Nerve damage affects 60 to 70 percent of diabetics in the form of numbness, tingling sensations or a loss of feeling in a diabetic's extremities especially the feet. As a matter of fact diabetic leg ulcer or un-healing foot wounds are a result of poor circulation and the person is unable to feel the pain because of neuropathy and can end up with a limb amputated.

Germany is one of the countries in the world that spends excessive amounts of money in Complementary Alternative Medicine. Over the past 30 years Germany has conducted several double blind studies using 300 to 600 mg a day of Alpha-lipoic acid in successfully treating neuropathy.[128] Alpha-lipoic acid has also been shown to lower high glucose levels.

The B vitamins are another set of nutrients that have shown promise in the elimination of neuropathy. Vitamin B6 has been noted for its ability to reduce carpel tunnel syndrome and in several studies it has been used to treat neuropathy. In a six-month research study conducted by Hayward, California Kaiser Permanente Medical Center, they administered 160 mg a day of vitamin B6 for chronic neuropathy pain. Their result was that the pain decreased, moods changed and their life activities increased and the hyperglycemia drugs were decreased.[129]

A 2 year research study conducted by the University of Manchester in England of 46 type 1 and type 2 diabetic patients ages 57 with chronic peripheral painful neuropathy used acupuncture as the form of treatment. The results of the study showed there was a 77% improvement in the diabetes and neuropathy of the 44 participant, who completed the study. The follow up showed the intake of diabetic medication was reduced by 67% and acupuncture was only requested by 24% of the patients. The symptoms of 21% of the diabetics were eliminated and one person complained of side effects.[130] [131]

The pain of neuropathy is consistent and diabetics are always looking for relief. Cayenne pepper, also known as capsaicin (Capsicum frutescens) aids in the reduction of neuropathy pain. Capsaicin has shown to relieve 80 percent of the diabetic neurological pain.[132] When applied to the skin cayenne is able to block pain of the nervous system and joints from reaching the brain.

One of the undiscovered micronutrients that I found to work well for neuropathy is CoEnzyme Q10. In a case study I will share with you later my finding of the use of 200 mg a day of Co Q10 that assisted in the reduction and elimination of the pain, tingling and numbness associated with neuropathy. In the long term neuropathy did not return, however, there needs to be more research on this to conclude the usefulness of Q10 as a clinical application for neuropathy. As we know, Q10 maintains the balance of the mitochondria of the cells building the energy force of the cell including the nervous cell.

Wound Healing and Foot Ulcers

"The healthier the blood, the greater the vitality and longer the span of life. For it is the quality of the blood which determines the strength of our bones and the firmness of our muscles."

Ann Wigmore
The Wheatgrass Book

Diabetes is also a disease of the circulatory system, causing increases or decreases of the flow of nutrients through the body, especially the lower limbs where it adversely affects the healing process for foot ulcers and wounds. Many diabetics can't heal foot ulcers due to a lack of blood supply to lower extremities and nerve degeneration. In advanced stages this failure to heal can transform unhealed wounds into gangrene where the person's foot or leg has to be amputated. The decrease of vital nutrients such as vitamin C and zinc are key elements in the ability to heal and both are deficient in diabetics. By increasing the dosage of both, as discussed in the protocol, the wounds will heal.

In my center I have suggested the use of Aloe Vera gel on the extremity (not in the open wound), as well as the consumption of 2 ounces of pure aloe twice a day (African Aloe Vera) for five days each week.

Aloe has shown to be an anti-inflamitive, herb promoting the normalization of blood sugar levels and increasing the ability of the body to absorb nutrients. As a wound healer, scientific studies have shown the active ingredients in aloe to activate immunity and increase the macrophage process of fighting infections and bacteria as it repairs the cellular structure. Its ability to increase wound healing has to do with Aloe's promotion of oxygenation to the blood and cells.

Because I am a traditional Chinese Herbalist, my formulation, are to increase the circulation of Qi (energy) and blood into the lower extremities, consist of herbs that reduce heat, increase the flow of blood and Qi. These herbs are consumed for five days each week on an empty stomach. Over the years I have seen my formulation not only improve the circulation in the lower extremities, but improve the energy levels and complexion of the person as well as increase their ability to heal more rapidly from any injury.

Eye Disease Susceptible to Diabetes

"By consciously building the type of physical body that is able to be sensitive to, attract, conduct, nurture, and hold the higher spiritualizing energies, we become more capable of holding the full power of God's Light."

Gabriel Cousens, M.D.
Conscious Eating

Eye disease is common with diabetics including Cataracts, Glaucoma, and Retinopathy, which can lead to blindness. Any unusual eye issues (floating spots, redness, blurred vision, or pressure) diabetics experience should be checked by their physician and they should have an eye exam at lest once a year.

Cataracts

Cataracts cause vision to become cloudy because they block light from penetrating the lens of the eye. According to the American Diabetic Association, diabetics are 60 percent more likely to have cataracts then non-diabetics. Cataracts are responsible for the blindness of 40,000 Americans each year. Studies have shown that a lack of antioxidants and the growth of free radicals can be responsible for cataracts.[133]

In the book "Natural Cures" it states: "We now know that senile cataracts are caused by damage from free radicals, the unbalanced, destructive molecules that destroy cells in the body." It went on to comment about cataracts being a nutritional deficiency, when it stated, "Poor digestive function can be at the root of cataracts. Low stomach acid can lead to mal-absorption of nutrients from foods and can create more free radicals.[134] [135] [136]

Harvard University conducted a study with 110,000 men and women using foods high in antioxidants to determine the affects of the antioxidants lutein and zeaxanthin on the development of cataracts. The results of the study showed when people consume dark green leafy vegetables full of carotenoids at lest three times a week it protects their eyes.

In order for a diabetic to address cataracts they have to first work on stabilizing their blood sugar levels. Improve their eating habits and begin a regiment of antioxidants. Over the period of a week you should incorporate antioxidant rich foods such as beet greens, broccoli, collard greens, kale, and most all greens are good sources of antioxidants and caroteniods. All types of colorful fruits and vegetables should be consumed within the week, some of which should be eaten raw. You should take digestive enzymes to assist in the correcting the digestive tract more on this in the health and healing section. It is also good to reduce your red meat intake because of the increasing amounts of hormones, antibiotics, and abundant amount of archodonic acid. Learn different types of eye exercises to help strengthen the eye muscles and increase the blood flow to the eyes.

Glaucoma

Glaucoma is where the fluids in the eye are unable to drain and pressure builds in the eye eventually to the point of nerve and retina damages resulting in blindness. Diabetics are at a greater risk of developing glaucoma.

In traditional Chinese medicine the eyes are the sensory organs of the liver and when the liver's energy is stagnated or has created heat it will increase the pressure in the eyes and reducing the ability of the fluids to drain to the point where a person can suffer from glaucoma. The liver plays a role in the transformation of glycogen to glucose and where there is an excessiveness of liver energy then that transformation is unable to take place, which also can result in Glaucoma. In the Chinese medical section there is more discussion about the liver and its role in diabetes and health.

Studies show Alpha-lipoic acid (100-300 mg a day, take the dosage throughout the day.), Vitamin B1, vitamin B2, pantothenic acid, and vitamin B6 aid in the reduction of eye fluid (take 200/mg of each of the B vitamins with 200 mg of B complex). Magnesium not only lowers blood sugar levels, but also increases the fluid in the eyes by relaxing the blood vessels to the eyes. Throughout the day 900 mg should be taken with a meal along with 1,600 mg of calcium, 400 mg of vitamin D, and 3,000 mg of vitamin C (vitamin C should be taken in units of 1,000mg at a time for best absorption).

Retinopathy

Diabetic Retinopathy is when excessive amounts of sugar in the blood weaken small blood vessels of the eye, increasing blood vessels leakage of plasma and blood into the retina damaging it causing a loss of vision.

Retinopathy responses well to 3,000 mg of vitamin C (you should take 1,000 mg 3 times a day), foods that are high in bioflavenoids or take bioflavoniods capsules (250 mg). Success has been shown with Bilberry extract at 320 mg according to Dr. Michael Murray.

Stepping Into the Future With a Healthy Lifestyle Program

"When we first begin to work with Nature and all of its inherent energies, some tremendous benefits come to us."

Ted Andrews
Nature-Speak

The major cause of type 2-diabetes is impairment of a person's ability to eat foods and have them digest, absorb and assimilate and the waste by products expelled in a timely manner. Type 1 diabetes occurs with when a person's immune system is unable to maintain its ability to protect the person, which has to do with how well foods are processed in the body to aid in protecting the cells, tissues, and organs. We don't realize the nutrients from food create life's balances. Without it there is only air and water to live on and most people would have to really change their life style in order to be a breathiterian or fast all of their life. So, we have to say that food is essential in our life, even though we can live days without food.

If you are asking, *"What is missing in my ability to be well?"* the real question you should be asking is, *"How does what I eat affect my ability to maintain health and heal me from diabetes."* Once you answer that question you are on the road to healing. It is a simple question that has a lot of impact in the world of healing. The answer is also simple. Change your eating habits and your thought patterns, exercise and live life to it's fullest. This just means you will have to work for your health. It is something you have not done because you have diabetes and other complications. Look for the sweetness of your life and not all the sweets you can eat.

A healthy lifestyle change protocol introduces you to information that will assist you in eating healthy, balancing your meals, reducing cholesterol, lowering and/or eliminating both diabetes, and hypertension. You will lose weight along with eradicating all the complications that goes with diabetes. The protocol will assist you in increasing your nutritional values promoting and elevating your energy levels and allowing you to begin to live a life without diabetes. This protocol aids you in understanding what to eat, how to eat it and when to eat it, as well as which supplements to take and how to take them to aid in maintaining your health. This is not a temporary solution or a diet program; it is a life long change if you use the information.

This process requires you to change your mind set and have the will to want to change. I suggest if you are not ready for the change then you stop reading now. On the other hand, if you are serious about changing your lifestyle than you should read on and practice the methods suggested. I set this protocol up over 15 years ago and many people have had success in reducing and/or eliminating their diabetes and are living a healthy and wonderful life without the use of medication and in some cases without the herbal formulas for diabetes.

As I stated earlier the body is a chemistry factory and you are the chemist. Everything you consume, wear, think or touch promotes some type of chemical reaction. Each food and combination creates a chemical change and depending on the combination depends on how well the body will function after you eat. Food actually determines how well your body will heal and stay healthy. By using the method I set forth you will be able to see a difference in your weight, diabetes, cholesterol, hypertension and bowel function.

The information provides you with an understanding of the elements the body needs to maintain health and eliminate diabetes including: good fats and bad fats, carbohydrate and their usage, along with amino acids. I teach you how to combine foods for better digestion, explain methods of using the glycemic index and optimum diabetes prevention and/or elimination. The healthy lifestyle program introduces you to the biochemical relationship between food and your body. It offers the understanding of balance that is necessary for the body to heal.

In order to correct your issues with diabetes you will have to first relean how to eat, including the mastication process of chewing food well. Food must be chewed until it is liquid in your month creating a bolus of smaller digestible particles. This complete mastication assists in filling the food molecules with needed enzyme for digestion. Because diabetes is a multi digestive disorder complete mastication is imperative as well as the implementation of proteolytic enzymes therapy as part of their lifestyle changes. This therapy assists in the process of digestion, absorption, and assimilation to create proper elimination of waste by products from the foods consumed.

The next step in overcoming diabetes is to incorporate proper food combining techniques; allowing foods to be digested in the correct areas of the body for optimum absorption of nutrients from foods consumed. This means diabetics have to learn the interaction between the chemical mixture of their food and its ability to digest in the body. They have to understand that starches, proteins, sugars, and lipid (fats) do not mix well together and they will destabilize the gut flora resulting in immunity problems, leaky gut syndrome and other complications. You have to make a conscious effort to combine your foods well in order to increase nutritional values to reduce and/or eliminate nutritional deficiencies associated with diabetes. You have to understand drinking and eating at the same time can disrupt the digestive process resulting in food particles lodged in your small intestines for an extended period of time upset the delicate balance of gut flora reducing the absorption and assimilation of nutrients.

The multi-digestive disorder of diabetes creates Mal-absorption of nutrients resulting in Mal-nutrition. With Mal-absorption and Malnutrition being the underlining issues of both types of diabetes, micronutrient therapy is a must in correcting the nutritional deficiencies associated with diabetes. As a matter of fact evidence of these studies identifies micronutrients deficiencies as the major cause of both types of diabetes. By increasing the intake of micronutrients you are able to reduce and/or eliminate diabetes and its complications.

Micronutrients are minerals, vitamins, enzymes, amino acids and other nutrients assisting the body in its ability to promote health and well being. You should be able to receive them from the foods you eat, however there are many factors that reduce your chances of receiving them. Many times the full range of nutrients is not in the food because of processing or overcooking. Other times it is because food is either mixed in wrong combinations or gulped and not chewed properly. These micronutrients are important for daily health. Because your diabetes is a metabolic disorder, you have to supplement micronutrients to aid in the balance of foods you consume. It has been shown that diabetics are deficient in many micronutrients and in order to reduce the high glucose blood levels you have to increase your micronutrient levels.

This protocol addresses this imbalance and provides information that will assist in understanding the delicate balance of micronutrients that will assist in the improvement of blood glucose levels. The micronutrients work synergistically together to create a balance in the body and promote health and healing. Some of the micronutrients are water soluble, meaning they will enter the body and work within the body to increase the body's function and then be excreted through the urine and bowels. Another type of micronutrient is the fat soluble. Fat-soluble vitamins enter the body and align with the fatty tissue and the liver remaining in the body for a longer period of time. They can build up in the body when taken in excess.

There are other supplements like minerals, which the body can manufacture; however, there are some essential minerals the body is unable to manufacture. Minerals are the backbone of the body, because they constitute the framework of the body, the blood, bones, tissues, organs, healthy nervous function, muscle toning, energy production, growth, development, maturity, and assist the function of vitamins and other nutrients in the body. These salts are essential for the body to heal and function naturally.

Amino Acids are a vital part of nutrition needed by the body, they develop into proteins and are building blocks of the body. As building blocks when deficient the body is unable to heal and maintain health. The protocol will discuss fatty acids, carbohydrates, the glycemic index and other elements to balance blood sugar levels the nervous system and other systems.

Enzymes: The Chains of Life

Nourishing foods put a spring in you walk, clear your mind, and balance your emotions. What you eat affects your every waking and sleeping hours.

Molly Siple M.S., R.D.
Healing Foods for Dummies

Enzymes are a natural substance that carry out every chemical action and reaction in the body and are the primary functions of life, without enzymes there would be no existence. Science has identified more then 2,700 enzymes in the human body that play a vital role in the metabolic functions of cells, tissues, organs, hormones, blood, body fluids, fats, carbohydrates, sugars, minerals, vitamins and the prime function of the brain. They are the workaholics maintaining the body's homeostasis (the maintenance of relatively stable internal physiological conditions as body temperature or PH balance).

Enzymes are protein base molecules performing specific jobs in the body including digestion, absorption, and eliminations. They repair the body after trauma, detoxification of systems, and processes neurological and mental activities.

Enzymes assist the digestive tract through a chemical reaction to the particles of food or beverage consumed, whether it is protein, starch, or lipid. The process aids in the food particles be absorbable by the stomach and small intestines to provide nourishment to the blood, tissues, muscles, nerves, bones, and glands. Enzymes play a critical role in the aging process and determine whether the body is able to maintain health.

The National Enzyme Commission identifies enzymes by the elements they act upon and place "ease" at the end of their name. For instance, protease synthesizes protein, lipase break down fats; cellulase synthesizes cellulose, amylase breaks down starch and maltase digests sugar. Some enzymes do not carry ease in their name like trypsin and pepsin.

The consumption of raw and fermented foods (sauerkraut, miso, tofu, etc, which are pre-digestible) provide their own enzymes, which assist in the digestive process. Eating these types of foods replenish the body's enzymes aiding in the maintenance and well being of the body. When foods are cooked and consumed the body is burdened with producing enough of its own enzymes to digest the food, which depletes the body's supply. In most cases our food is either overcooked or processed, which kills the enzymes. During a meal of cooked food, you should take digestive enzymes to assist in the digestion of the food and replenish the body's level of enzymes.

Enzymes are sensitive to heat and light. Enzymes decompose at a temperature of 118 degrees Fahrenheit. In their processing food manufacturers cook food well over 2,000 degrees Fahrenheit to reduce and/or eliminate the bacteria in food and then we cook them an additional 250 to 400 degrees Fahrenheit. At this point, there is no life giving properties left in the food. All the nutrients and enzymes have been destroyed and the food is a burden on the body. This causes weight gain, bowel problems and other health disparities. In children it can impede their growth and development.

When you eat processed, overcooked, chemical laced foods, the body has to produce its own enzymes in order to properly digest the foods, which means, if you have a health situation the body has to decide whether it will digest the food or continue to heal the body. If the body continues to heal its self, the food will not be digested. It then goes into the body and is stored as waste, contributing to obesity, overweight conditions, hypertension, diabetes and other health disparities.

On the other hand, when you eat processed food, the enzymes are *"dead"* with a minimal to no life giving properties. Frozen, prepackaged, cooked and canned foods are all enzymes deprived, with little or no nutrients. This could hold true also in foods that are laced with dyes, additives, preservative, pesticides and herbicides.

During disease our bodies' need for enzymes is greater. If there is a deficiency the body tries to receive nutrients from wherever it can, leaving some areas of the body depleted. In the replenishing state, the body will shut itself down, resulting in fatigue; muscle cramps, and overall body weakness. This is when you may feel tired in the middle of the day or right after exercising. In today's society 90% of the population feels tired almost all the time because the foods eaten are not digesting and the foods have no enzyme or other nutrients contributing to the body's wellness. These foods are causing the body to work harder and overtime to muster whatever energy it can. All of this food lacking nutrients has made way for people to look for energy in other place then the nourishment from food and manufacturers have accommodated us with all these energy drinks, shakes, and bars that not only have little to no nutrients, but are loaded with sugar.

We must understand our ancestors received their energy and nourishment from the foods they ate, which allowed their bodies to heal and grow strong. These enzyme rich foods would build cells, tissues, and organs and increase their brainpower. They had an abundance of energy and lived to ripe old ages over 100 years and their minds were sharp until they died. There was some diabetes and other health issues; however, it was not at epidemic levels as it is today.

Eating raw or partially cooked food provides the body with a greater amount of enzymes, which improves ones nutritional values. Raw fruits and vegetables contain an abundance of enzymes promoting and assisting the body in maintaining health and wellbeing. Enzymes in fruits and vegetables increase the body's chance of preventing and eliminating health conditions. Raw foods are also full of antioxidants, carotenes, phenols, carbohydrate, fats and sugars that work in harmony to increase health.

Digestion and absorption relies on enzymes to break down food into liquids for absorption and assimilation in the body. This is why it is important to chew (masticate) your food well. When we do not masticate our food well and it is swallowed in large pieces or eaten in the wrong combination, the enzyme **"amylolytic"** found in the alkaline environment of the mouth is unable to digest starch and carbohydrates. When proteins are consumed, which is a group of amino acids; they need protease a *"proteolytic"* enzyme to digest them in the acid environment of the stomach. If proteolytic enzymes are deficient and/or hydrochoric acid is deficent, proteins are unable to be digested. The protein moves into the small intestine where it putrefies and causes obstructions in the bowels. Without the absorption of protein, the body will have problems with growth and development.

Fats or lipids, which are triglycerides, phospholipids, and sterols, need *"lipolytic"* enzymes to assist in the decomposition of its structure. In cases where fats are present but there is a lack of lipases to break them down, they lodge in other areas of the body, such as in the blood as cholesterol, or in the adipose tissues as fat. An imbalance of lipolytic enzymes results in high cholesterol, weight gain, cardiovascular disease, and other health conditions.

Many people with diabetes have polyuria (excessive urination) that also can lead to protein in the urine. It is easy to spot this because the urine has a lot of bubbles. This could be caused by an infection or other kidney imbalances. It is safe to consult your physician who will offer test to determine where it is coming from. It has not been diagnosed as, but it can be looked at as an enzyme deficiency that reduces the kidneys ability to store and maintain the proper protein levels. Enzyme therapy has been known to reduce and/or eliminate the protein in your urine. In my experience I have worked with diabetics who have had this issue and by increasing the amount of metabolic enzymes consumed eliminated the protein in their urine. Someday researchers will identify enzyme deficiency as a major issue in health disparities.

Sugar, which is a disaccharide is digested by disacchardases and converted into glucose for the body to use as energy. When disacchardases is deficient sugars are unable to be digested resulting in high blood glucose levels.

Sugar is one of the major foods eaten in the United States. It is stated that American's consume a 150 pounds of sugar a year. On the other hand, when people have an intolerances to sugar they consume more protein because 40% of the usable protein is converted to energy.

The Life of Carbohydrates

"Human beings, the culmination of billions of years of natural evolution, are formed from the dynamic interaction of heaven's and earth's forces."

Michio Kushi and Alex Jack
The Macrobiotic Path to Total Health

Carbohydrates are the staples of life and yet society has classified them as a dangerous food that contributes to all types of unhealthy conditions including weight gain, obesity, hypertension, diabetes, cardiovascular disease, etc. There is some truth to this statement because the majority of the carbohydrates being consumed are refined starches and processed sugars. It is not the carbohydrates per say causing weight gain and other health conditions, but the refining process striping all of the nutrients from the carbohydrates.

The interesting thing is that when manufacturers process grains and cereals, the essences of these foods are lost. Due to the law manufacturers have to replace them with synthetic nutrients known as "enrichment". The synthetic nutrients are unable to be absorbed in the body, impairing digestion, absorption and elimination, resulting in an accumulation of waste in the small intestine. Because of the health issues posed by refined carbohydrates medical society has issued a low or no carbohydrate campaign that has many people convinced that they should stay away from carbohydrates because they are a health risk. This is why we are witnessing high protein diets.

Carbohydrates are energy foods assisting in maintaining health and immunity. Carbohydrates are comprised of carbon, hydrogen and oxygen molecules, which are the major elements of the human body; without which the body would disintegrate back into the earth from which it came.

Most carbohydrates are plant-based products with the ability to receive photosynthesis from the sun. The sun packs them full of life given nutrients that humans are unable to directly receive from the sun. Humans should receive 85 to 90% of their carbohydrates from plant life and the remainder from dairy products (which many people have an intolerants to). We find carbohydrates in the forms of grains, sugars, vegetables, fruits, beans, peas and cereals. Eating carbohydrates in their natural unprocessed state the body's amylolytic enzymes are able to digest them and use them as fuel. On the other hand, when adulterated (processed) carbohydrates are consumed, they lack the nutritional values and produce empty calories, which stores in the body as fat and increase sweet and sugar carving to maintain our energy levels. Many people who are heavy protein eaters also crave sweets because of the lack of energy they receive from the excessive proteins. It is interesting that the same Dr. Fredrick Banting who discovered insulin also started the first concept of a high protein diet being good for people. We have been led to believe that Dr. Akins was the first. Banting found that people would lose weight but gain cholesterol problems. These sweets can come in the form of fruits or hidden sugars in meats and other products eaten. The calorie-conscious high protein eaters stay within their limits of carbohydrates.

Carbohydrates are "saccharum," the Latin word for sugar. They are classifications by size and water solubility, which governs how well they will work in the body. Monosaccharides have the smallest molecule chain and are very soluble in water. They are comprised of glucose, fructose, galactose, xylose, mannose and ribose. There are over 100 different types of monosaccharides in nature. As a matter of fact, carbohydrates are the most abundant compound in nature and consumed by every mammal in the universe. All vegetarian animals consume carbohydrates in their natural form without a risk of obesity; yet humans become obese from carbohydrates. Many of these animal are big and have energy to spare like the gorillas and giraffes and throughbred horses running at speeds of 40 miles per hour, they eat carbohydrates yet they don't get diabetes. Horses chew on wood sometimes because of nutritional deficiencies. Experienced trainers understand the issues and provide them with nutrients (vitamins, minerals, etc) to correct the problem. It is amazing that society would take better care of lower animals than itself.

The other thing is that these animals take their time eating their food and chew it well, mixing the enzymes in their mouths with the food to enhance the digestive process. Humans eat on the run, under stress, and gulp the food down, not chewing enough so that the food skips the enzyme breakdown process that should occur in the mouth.

Disaccharides, on the other hand, have two sugar molecules in the form of sucrose (sugar cane, beet, maltose, and lactose) that is extracted from grains and animal milk. In the case of polysaccharides, which have 12 or more monosaccharides, they are in the form of cellulose, inulin and other non-flexible chains that are not as water-soluble.

Polysaccharides are comprised of the compound chondroitin sulfate, which is the major constituent of the body's cartilage tissues. Polysaccharides provide energy in the form of starches and glycogen in mammals' bodies. Oligosaccharide is comprised of two to ten monosaccharide chains (raffinose and stachyose) that affect the digestive tract in general.

In order for the body to maintain its' DNA and RNA levels, it has to have carbohydrates in the form of ribose, which is manufactured in the cells from glucose. Gylcosomin chondroitin is the by-product of glycosaminoglycans (GAGs), a complex carbohydrate that promotes the fluid motion that reduces or possibly eliminates joint pain and inflammation.

The stories of carbohydrates dates back to ancient civilization where carbohydrates like oats were not only used as food, but also as medicine. Carbohydrates are the major food groups of many cultures of the world. Many rely on carbohydrates in the form of rice, beans and grains to maintain life. The carbohydrates eaten by these cultures are not adulterated. It is interesting that whenever there is a national disaster or when the world feed refugees or other displaced starving people they are always given carbohydrates in the form of grains. It would make you wonder why society is telling us carbohydrates are bad for us to eat.

It is not the carbohydrates that are the major cause of being overweight or obese; it is the process by which they are being manufactured and how we are consuming them. The carbohydrates are being refined with all the nutrients and enzymes being striped away leaving nothing but empty calories that are indigestible. The processing of carbohydrates depletes the B vitamins, enzymes and other essential elements found in grains, beans, vegetables and sugars, which are needed if they are to be digested and absorbed in the body for increasing and maintaining health. The natural fibers of these processed foods are also eliminated and cannot be replaced synthetically like other nutrients, which results in the accumulation of waste byproducts in the small intestine causing constipation, gas, cardiovascular disease, bowel problems and other health disparities.

When wastes byproducts of carbohydrates accumulate in the small intestine, they begin to distend the abdomen. This distention is the small intestine expanding to accommodate an excessive amount of waste accumulating within its' walls. This excessive accumulation begins to leak into the blood (leaky gut syndrome) further causing the carbohydrate waste-by-products to also store in the adipose tissues (fat cells) resulting in weight gain. This increase of adipose tissue begins creating obstructions in the blood vessels and throughout the organ network.

Glycoproteins, which are saccharides linked to proteins, are another source of abdominal distention, accumulation of waste, and the leaky gut syndrome. When this starch and protein combinations does not digest in the body it putrefies and ferments resulting in unhealthy bowel conditions that lead to other health disparities.

There are two types of carbohydrates—complex and simple. Complex carbohydrates include grains, legumes, and vegetables. These are foods that do not have a sweet taste and are mostly starches with an abundance of minerals, vitamins, amino acids, enzyme, etc. On the other hand, simple carbohydrates are sugars and do have a sweet taste, which include sucrose, sugars and fruits. When sweeteners are added to grains, (which are bad combinations) it changes the structure of the carbohydrate from a complex carbohydrate to a simple carbohydrate such as cakes, cookies, pies, etc. Because of their many monosaccharide chains, complex carbohydrates are further divided into high and low fiber categories.

When complex carbohydrates are processed they break down like simple carbohydrates and attack the body in the same manner. When the germ is stripped from the wheat and turned to white flour this new product has the ability to cause disease. White flour as I have stated earlier has an element called alloxan, which causes diabetes. These processed grains lose all of their vital nutrients, which is why these products have to be enriched with synthetic nutrients. The synthetic nutrients are difficult for many people to digest and absorb, so they begin to have an allergic reaction to the products. This is when the body is unable to process the product, thus increasing the histamine protein, causing the body to cough, sneeze, eyes to water and causing nasal drip. This is what we refer to as an allergy and a person reaches for anti-histamines to control the problem. Processed carbohydrates also increase blood glucose levels.

Fiber is one of the main components of complex carbohydrates. It helps move the bowels and prevent colon cancer and other diseases. Dietary fiber also has an impact on diabetes and hypertension. These groups of polysaccharides are indigestible and include a variety of foods such as almonds, wheat germ, psyllium seed and husk, beans, rice, barley, apples, green vegetables, etc. It is recommended by the World Health Organization (WHO) that each person should consume 25 to 40 grams of fiber daily. Most Americans only receive 12 to 18 grams a day. Humans need to incorporate plant fiber in their daily regimens because most of us eat indigestible foods that cause health disparities. Dr. Bernard Jensen once said, "Death begins in the colon."

Your eating habits should consist of enough fruits, vegetables and grains to provide the nutrients and fiber needed to maintain good nutrition and positive bowel evacuation in a timely manner. Too much fiber can cause problems of bloating, gas, and abdominal cramping. Whenever you consume substances like bran or psyllium, you should drink two to three 8-ounce glasses of water. If the fiber is not well lubricated, it can cause a host of bowel problems. Most vegetables, fruits and whole grains have a large amount of fiber that will increase the peristaltic process of the colon. As I have pointed out, constipation is one of the many issues affecting diabetics. By increasing your vegetables, legumes, beans, nuts, seeds and some fruits, you will witness bowel regularity, lower blood sugars, and a reduction in weight.

The Dance of the Maze (Body Mass Index, Glycimic Index, Glycimic Load)

"Problem solving is one of the great joys of the practice of medicine, particularly when the solution enriches the life of a sick person in the process."

Larry Dossey, M.D.
Healing Beyond the Body

The concept for the Glycemic Index came out of a research project carried out by David Jenkins, M.D., and his colleagues at the University of Toronto, Canada. They evaluated how quickly the body would metabolize glucose from each food consumed, basing it on the consumption of white bread. The importance of the Glycemic Index (GI) is to show how rapidly certain foods increase the blood sugar level at the conversion of 50 to 100 grams of glucose in these foods. The calculation of a low GI is 55, moderate GI is 56-69 and high GI is 70 to 100. High GI foods cause blood sugar levels to spike, increasing the amount of glucose rapidly entering the blood stream and increasing the output of insulin. On the other hand, low glycemic foods release glucose at a slower rate where the cells are able to uptake the glucose without a major increase of insulin.

The glycemic index was surrounded by controversy because of the area of the world where the food was grown, its processing methods and preparation, as well as food combining, the amount of food consumed and the differences in each person's metabolism. For instance oatmeal has a GI of 48 whereas cream of wheat is 66 and cornflakes are at 83. In this example Oatmeal will absorb in the blood easier, cornflakes will increase the blood sugar levels more and it may be more difficult for the cells to absorb the glucose. Evidence has recently showed the consumption of a low GI diet will reduce the risk of developing obesity,[137] [138] colon cancer[139] and breast cancer. [140]

Glycemic Load

The glycemic load is the numerical calculation of the amount of carbohydrates in a food in conjunction with the glycemic index. Depending on this calculation will determine the effect a food has on the blood sugar and how quickly the glucose will enter the cells. Proper food combining is very important in the GL because, depending on which other foods you eat with carbohydrates, it will determine whether the carbohydrate will stabilize or increase blood sugar levels, then how high will the levels go before the blood accepts the glucose. For instance, starches and proteins are incompatible; however, in the case of a diabetic they are compatible because of the protein's ability to reduce the increase of glucose in the body when they are consumed with carbohydrates. Together they will have a moderate to low release of glucose in the blood, reducing the ability for the blood sugar to elevate.

Refined foods are high on the glycemic index because the natural essences of the food have been striped away and there is nothing but pure starch or sugar in the product, which works to increase the blood sugar levels. Studies have shown that a longtime consumption of foods with high glycemic loads increase the prevalence of type 2 diabetes and cardiovascular disease. [141]

Glycemic Index Table

Low Glycemic		Low to moderate		Moderate to high		High	
Apple	38	Apricots Jam	55	Apricots canned	64	Bagels	72
Apple juice	41	Blueberry muffins	59	Bananas	62	Beets	

Agave nectar juice	11	Bran Chex	58	Cakes Angel Food	67	Candy	
Apricots dried	30	Bran muffins	60	Cantaloupe	65	Cheerios	74
All Bran cereal	44	Brown rice	59	Cream of wheat	66	Corn bran	75
Baby lima beans	32	Carrots		Cornmeal	68	Corn Chex	83
Banana bread	47	Danish	59	Couscous	65	Croissant	67
Barley	22	Honey	58	Figs		Corn flakes	83
Beans		Kiwi	52	Flour white		Crispix	87
Berries		Mango	55	Macaroni & cheese	64	Dark Rye bread	76
Black beans	30	Muesli Cereal	60	Nutri Grain	66	Dates dried	103
Bran Rice cereal	19	Orange juice	55	Pita bread		Graham crackers	74
Bread (sprouted)		Papaya	58	Potatoes (sweet and white)		Kaiser rolls	73
Broccoli		Peas		Pineapples		Millet	75
Buckwheat	54	Peaches		Rye crackers	63	Pies	
Bulger wheat	47	Potato chips		Shortbread cookies	64	Pretzels	
Butter beans	31	Pound cake	54	Grapenuts cereal	67	Parsnips	
Cashews		Special K	54	Raisins	64	Pasta brown Rice	92
Cherries	22	Whole Rye bread	50	Rye	64	Puff Wheat (cereal)	74
Chickpeas	36			Shredded Wheat	69	Rice white instant	91
Corn sweet	55			Wheat Thins (Stone Ground)	67	Rice cakes	82
Frosted Flakes	55					Rice Chex cereal	89
Grapes	43					Rice Krispies cereal	82
Grapefruit	25					Saltine crackers	72
Grapefruit juice	48					Total	76
Green leafy vegetables						Waffle	76
Ice cream	50					Water	
Kidney beans	27					Vanilla Wafers cookies	77
Lentil	30					Water crackers	78
Macaroni	46					Watermelon	72

Milk	34					Wheat pasta	
Milk chocolate	34						
Milk soy	31					Wheat Puff Rice	90
Navy	38					White bread	72
Orange	43					White rice	88
Oatmeal	49					Whole wheat bread	72
Oatmeal cookies	55						
Pasta (whole wheat)							
Peach	42						
Pears	36						
Pineapple juice	46						
Pinto beans	42						
Plums	24						
Pudding	43						
Pumpernickel bread	49						
Rye	34						
Rice white Parboiled	47						
Soybeans	18						
Sponge cake	46						
Split peas	32						
Strawberries	32						
Strawberry jam	51						
Wheat whole	41						
Tomatoes							
Wild rice							
Plain yogurt	38						

If a diabetic learns to properly combine foods with the aide of the food-combining chart, and to eat according to the glycemic index chart, they will find that their blood sugar levels decrease. When they incorporate the use of micronutrients and phytonutrients, their blood sugar levels will stabilize to the point where their AC1a hemoglycous exam will have a positive reading.

The major objective is to lower and stabilize blood sugar levels by incorporating the proper carbohydrates and eliminate starches and sugars that elevate blood sugar levels. It does not matter which type of sugar you intake; it will increase your blood sugar levels. White sugar digests the same as honey, high-fruit sugar and other types of sugar. All of them raise blood sugar levels. Sugars come in several different forms and are known by a variety of names, including barley malt syrups, blackstrap molasses, brown rice syrup, cane sugar, corn syrup, fructose, high corn fructose, honey, lactose, maltose, mannitol, maple syrup, rice syrup, saccharin, sorbitol sorghum, and sucrose.

High fructose is one of the sweeteners that many people gravitate to in replacing sugar. However, it is one of the most dangerous foods we can consume because it is the cause of obesity, diabetes, cancer and other health disparities. It has been known to increase glycosylation where it destroys protein at a higher rate than sucrose. Artificial sweeteners are not an advantage either; they have been linked to headaches, vision loss, seizures, nervous disorders, and mood swings. The majority of artificial sweeteners are made from chemicals; some don't have any sugar at all. That is why there are side effects and in some cases they have been linked to cancer.

While on my protocol, I have diabetics to stay clear of all types of sugar for the first 60 to 90 days. Their carbohydrate intake is low and their intake of fresh non-starches vegetables is high. If they need to have a sweetener that does not raise their blood sugar, I suggest Stevia, which is a subtropical herb grown in South America. Even though this herb is 15 times sweeter than cane sugar; it has almost no calories, and is promising in strengthening the cardiovascular and digestive systems. [142] Studies show it to be safe for diabetics to take without an elevation in their blood sugar levels.[143]

Contribution of Essential Fatty Acids

"Fat has become a foul three-letter word in our society. We've become a nation of fat phobics, and some of us try to avoid this nutrient at all costs in an effort to lose weight and improve our health. yet this war on fat has been completely misguided."

Dr. Barry Sears
The Omega R Zone

The body cannot live without fatty acids. Fatty acids are what we have always called fats, which are also known as lipids. Different types of fatty acids perform different tasks in the body. Some fatty acids are instrumental in the production of hormones, cholesterol, mobilizing joints, maintaining the pressure in the eyes, body tissue respiration, maintaining the balance of the immune system, dilating and distributing the pressure in the blood vessels, neurotransmission of the nervous system, maintenance of proper kidney function, preventing and protecting against cardiovascular disease, diabetes, cancer, autoimmune diseases, skin diseases, and chronic disease. As part of their work in the body, fatty acids synthesize bile, fat-soluble vitamins, and steroids. In other words, some fats maintain the health of the body.

These fatty acids are known as Essential Fatty Acids. Fats, whether oils, lards or waxes, are members of the lipid family. They are derived from animals, plants or microbial cells and are not soluble in water. Animal fat is saturated fat, while some vegetable oils are liquid polyunsaturated fat. Both are hydrocarbons comprised of hydrogen, carbon, and oxygen, which are related to the petroleum atoms. Cholesterol, on the other hand, is known as lipoproteins, which are monoglycerides.

The hydrocarbon chain making up lipids are comprised of three major fat groups; triglycerides, phospholipids, and steroids. Triglycerides are the bond between three fatty acids and glycerol molecules. These glycerol's develop into a triglyceride or natural fat, which are broken down during digestion into free flowing fatty acids. At that point they can be absorbed by the small intestine into the blood stream. After entering the blood, these triglycerides either work effectively to aid the body in maintaining health as healthy fats or they accumulate in the blood vessels, obstructing the walls of the vessels and causing unhealthy conditions.

About 95 percent of all the fat humans consume today are either saturated or unsaturated triglycerides. Whether a fatty acid is saturated or polyunsaturated depends on the amount of hydrogen atoms within the carbon chain. The chain is comprised of a double bond of carbon and hydrogen atoms, and any fat chain filled with hydrogen atoms is considered a saturated fat. On the other hand, a low amount of hydrogen atoms in a fatty acid chain makes it a polyunsaturated fatty acid.

When a fat is saturated it will be semisolid or solid at room temperature. When it is unsaturated it will be liquid at room temperature. When a person consumes an abundance of saturated fatty acids and a low amount of essential fatty acids (EFA's will be discussed in the next chapter) they have a greater risk of type 2 diabetes and other health conditions. Since the early part of the century, saturated fatty acid consumption in the United States has increased by 40 percent from 125 grams a day to 175 grams a day, increasing the prevalence of degenerate diseases.[144] The saturated fatty acids reduce the fluidity of the cell membrane reducing insulin's ability to bind to receptor cells.[145]

Triglycerides are stored in the fatty tissues (adipose) and meet the body's need for energy in between meals. When triglycerides are not immediately used after a meal they are converted to fat and stored in the adipose tissue at which point they can become excessive and turn into hypertriglyceridemia (insulin residents and high levels of triglycerides in the blood). Triglycerides need the enzyme lipase to properly digest into the system and build the body. If for any reason the small intestine is unable to digest the triglyceride then it will show up in the blood stream in the form of low-density lipoproteins (bad cholesterol).

Fats that are used or stored can also come from carbohydrates, which are first used for energy and then triglycerides. There are many cases where the accumulations of triglycerides in the adipose tissues are from refined carbohydrates and simple sugars. The accumulation of triglycerides in adipose tissues increase the risk for several diseases including diabetes mellitus, high cholesterol, coronary artery disease, cardiovascular disease, hypertension and other diseases. Ninety percent of the 60 to 150 grams of fats that an adult consumes a day are triglycerides. The reminder is comprised of cholesterol, cholesteryl esters, phospholipids, and free fatty acids. [146]

There are several other fatty acids including Stearic acid, Oleic acid (Omega 9), Linoleic, Gamma Linolenc acids (Omega 6), and Alpha-linoleic (Omega 3). These fatty acids are known as Omega oils and are essential fatty acids assisting the body in the production of prostaglandins (hormone-like substances).

These fatty acids are discussed under the section "Essential Fatty Acids." Oils, which are also fatty acids, are divided into cooking and medical oils. The latter oils are more heat sensitive then the cooking oils. Medical oils comprising the gamma-linolenic acid family include Black Currant oil, Oil of Borage, and Evening Primrose. Flax Seed is a medical oil of the alpha-linolenic fatty acid family. These oils are consumed through our eating habit in order for the body to utilize their nutritional values.

Vegetable cooking oils on the other hand have a higher tolerance for heat and can be used for cooking. However, too high temperatures destroy the molecular structure of the oil. This causes it to become dangerous to the body and increases the risk of developing into low-density lipoproteins (bad cholesterol). The best fatty acids for cooking are oleic fatty acids including canola oil and olive oil because they have a higher tolerance to heat as monounsaturated fatty acids.

When polyunsaturated oils like corn, safflower and soy oils are heated to high temperatures, they tend to become damaged quickly and their chemical structure changes, resulting in lipid peroxides.[147] Lipid peroxidation is the oxidative destruction of lipids resulting in the development of free radicals, which damage human blood cells causing cancer and other degenerative diseases.[148] At the same time it can also increase the level of cholesterol.

For years we have heard about Saturated and Polyunsaturated Fatty Acids and how one is a good fat and the other is a bad fat. The ironic thing is that just when we have begun to really understand the difference between saturated and polyunsaturated fats, we are introduced to harmful affects of Trans Fatty Acids (TFA). There is still a lot of research required to truly understand the working of TFA's in the body. The majority of TFA's are consumed through baked goods, snacks, crackers, cookies, cakes, potato chips, margarine, and shortening. To a lesser degree TFA's are found in animal products. Other TFA consumption comes from oils that are hydrogenated and excessively heated, like oils in fast food restaurants. As of January 2006, the law requires food manufactures to list on the label the total amount of TFA's in their products.

According to the American Heart Association, "*Trans* fats (or *trans* fatty acids) are created in an industrial process that adds hydrogen to liquid vegetable oils to make them more solid. Another name for *Trans* fats is "partially hydrogenated oils."[149] Trans fatty acids are cheap to make and can be used for a long period of time. TFA have been linked to elevated cholesterol, strokes, high blood pressure, overweight, obesity and type 2 diabetes. Trans fatty acids are hydrogenated which interfere with the metabolic process. They also impair the liver and gallbladders' ability to synthesize, secrete bile salts and convert high-density lipoproteins into free fatty acid in order to be absorbed by the small intestine. TFA's elevate Low Density Lipoproteins (LDL) bad cholesterol and lower High Density Lipoproteins (HDL) good cholesterol. Cholesterol has already been discussed.

Essential Fatty Acids

There are dozens of scientifically plausible ways food can affect health. However, three umbrella theories fuel and shape much new research into food's healing and preventive powers.

* *Disease-fighting antioxidants in foods*

* *The unappreciated pharmacological power of fat*

* *New kinds of food "allergies" or intolerances.*

Jean Carper
Food your Miracle Medicine

Essential Fatty Acids (EFA) are a good, healthy fat the body needs to perform several different functions, however, the body is unable to manufacture EFA's so we have to receive them through our eating habit. They are known for lowering cholesterol, reducing elevated blood pressure and assisting in the rebalancing of blood glucose levels.[150] Omega 3 and 6 are both EFAs that provide the body with different types of nutrients. Together they comprise prostaglandins, hormone-like substances that assist in temperature regulations, glandular functions, and the coagulation of the blood.

EFAs are important for the conversion of Linoleic and Linolenic acids into prostaglandins, which are hormone-like substances that maintain the blood's ability to clot, the stability of blood pressure, cell platelet aggregation, gastrointestinal secretions and function, kidney fluid balance and function, and transmission of neurological signaling. Prostaglandins are also responsible for the production of steroids and the synthesizing of hormones. They decrease the prevalence of swelling, pain and inflammation.

The increased consumptions of saturated fatty acids (arachidonic acid found in animal food products) with the insufficiency of essential fatty acids destabilize blood cells causing the cells not to respond to insulin signaling that link to type 2 diabetes.[151] EFAs assists cells in maintaining their integrity of electrolyte stability, water balance, and vital nutrients. Studies indicate the consistent consumption of omega 3 fatty acids improves cells uptake of glucose as it promote insulin activities preventing type 2 diabetes.[152]

Omega 3 Fatty Acids is oil from cold water fish including cod, mackerel, salmon, herring, sardines, tuna, white fish, etc as well as flax seeds, hemp seeds and also found in organ meat and eggs comprised of Alpha-Linolenic Acid, EicosaPentanic Acid (EPA), and Docosa Hexaenoic Acid (DHA). It aids in the regulations of neurocircuits, fatty acids of the brain, and the development of the retina of the eye (eye problems and blindness are complications of diabetes). In it's conversion to Gamma Linolenic Acid, which assists in the development of cholesterol lowering lipoproteins that also decrease triglycerides and decreases excessive blood fat as it promotes a healthy metabolism and blood composition. The composition of Omega 3 fatty acid reduces high blood pressure, decreases the prevalence of cardiovascular disease and atherosclerosis, which are all complications of diabetes. When taking omega 3 you should also incorporate vitamins C and E for best absorption. Omega 3 is found in most all vegetables oils (Canola and Olive oil) and nut oils (walnuts). The best source of omega 3 is fish oil, flaxseed and hemp oil. Other sources are anchovies, chia seeds, dark leafy green vegetables, and Spirulina (sea algae).

Omega 6 is another fatty acid that the body does not manufacture and is taken to maintain healthy cholesterol levels. It reduces the prevalence of cardiovascular disease, hardening of the arteries, atherosclerosis and is needed for healthy brain and nervous system functions (diabetics often have neuropathy tingling and numbness of the extremities). It maintains and balances glandular hormonal functions (thyroid, adrenals, etc.). All of which are part of diabetes complications. Gamma Linolenic acid (GLA), which is the Omega 6 fatty acid, is 10 times more active than Linolenic acid making it very valuable in cell growth and development.

Its blood vessel opening vassal dilation is powerful when consumed in conjunction with zinc. Omega 6 fatty acid also increases the activity of the immune system, which can assist type 1 diabetics in reducing their immune systems attack on the alpha and beta cell distortion. It influences the proper function of the heart reducing and obstruction that may cause cardiovascular disease, which is a cousin to diabetes. For the best absorption also take with vitamin C and B6. Most all vegetables and nut oils have omega 6 fatty acids. The best Omega 6 fatty acids are black currant oil, borage oil, evening primrose, and grape seed oils. Omega 6 fatty acids are also found in meat. Most people receive an excess of omega 6 fatty acids because of the amount of meat that is consumed. The excess of omega 6 fatty acid in many cases causes a uric acid build up in the joint promoting arthritis.

GLA is of the Omega 6 fatty acid type that has the ability to convert to Arachidonic acid (animal fat) and when it converts from Gamma-linolenic acid to Di-homo-gamma-linolenic acid (DHGLA) it develops into type 2 prostaglandin. This type of prostaglandin leads to cardiovascular disease, hardening of the arteries, stroke and blood platelet stickiness. Where in the GLA prostaglandins form of 1 and 3, it improves over all health conditions. Prostaglandins 2 are detrimental to health without the assistance of 1 and 3 found in Omega 3 fatty acids. This is why Omega 6 should be taken with Omega 3 and 9. The mixture of the three oils should come from vegetable oils and not have a mixture with fish oil. Fish oils should be taken separately from vegetable and seed oils.

The ratio of Omega 6 to 3 is for every 4 ounce of Omega 6 there should be 1 ounce of Omega 3 oil. In this society the ratio is more like 20 to 1, especially amongst meat eaters. I suggest my clients take Omega 3, 6, and 9 together or just take a tablespoon of Omega 3 for 5 days each week. I have found that when diabetics take either 4 capsules a day of Nortic Natural or Total EFA's it works well to improve the blood glucose levels and reduce the prevalence of atherosclerosis.

Omega 9 is not an essential fatty acid, however the body can manufacture and consume it through your eating habit, in the form of unsaturated fatty acids. In the body it aids in normalizing blood pressure, increasing metabolism, lowering cholesterol, improves mother's breast milk fatty acids, which can reduce a child's prevalence of type 1 diabetes.

Alpha-Lipoic Acid

Every beam of sunlight, every breath of fresh air, every drink of pure water, and every taste of living plant food takes us closer to the truth. These essencial nutrients contribute to the full circle of body, mind, and spirit.

Rita Romano
Dining in the RAW

Germany spent a great deal of time and money researching the affects of Alpha-Lipoic Acid on diabetes and it is used as an approved drug for diabetic neuropathy. In several of their studies they found that this antioxidant, vitamin-like substance is not manufactured by the body but is needed for several bodily functions. One of the major uses of alpha-lipoic acid in Europe was for nerve damage (peripheral neuropathy). The Diabetes Research Institute of Munich Germany held a symposium where they discussed the relationship between alpha-lipoic acid and diabetic neuropathy. What they found was that alpha-lipoic acid increased the uptake of glucose resulting in the decrease of neuropathy. Studies show, after administering 600 mg a day of ALA for 30 days orally to 10 polyneuropathy patients, that their neuropathy significantly improved and their blood flow increased. [153]

ALA also affects the Krebs Cycles where glucose is broken down into energy and cells are able to uptake glucose. It has been shown that ALA supplementation can prevent beta cell destruction, thus upsetting the prevalence of type 1 and type 2 diabetes. [154]

Frank Murray in his book Natural Supplements for Diabetes discussed how Russian researchers studied alpha-lipoic acid to treat heart disease and to reduce cholesterol. He presented a study where 38 type 2 diabetics and cardiac autonomic neuropathy patients were given a daily dose of 800 mg of alpha-lipoic acid, along with 34 patients that were given a placebo for a period of four months. The conclusion: the administration of alpha-lipoic acid reduced peripheral neuropathy and improved cardiac functions.[155]

As an antioxidant, alpha-lipoic acid improves the uptake of glucose and increases insulin sensitivity, because of its ability to improve the quality and life extension of vitamins C and E, which both are deficient in diabetics and have an impact on glucose levels.

Lecithin, The Cell Protector

"Although health has always been one of mankind's main concerns, most people aren't very interested in learning how to keep themselves healthy. it seems that we don't really appreciate our health until we lost it."

DR. Yang, Jwing-Ming
Qigong Massage

Lecithin, the cell protector, every cell in the body needs lecithin. It is the sheath surrounding the nerves, muscles and especially the brain. Lecithin is an interesting substance because it is a lipid (fat), yet it is water-soluble. This makes it a substance that has the ability to act as an emulsifier (it can break down fat and wax). It has the power to mix water and lipids together as one substance allowing the lipids to break down and be moved through the body. It also aids the body in absorbing fat-soluble vitamins like vitamins A, D, E, and F (essential fatty acids).

Lecithin is found in soybeans and egg yolks. Other sources of lecithin include brewer's yeast, grains, legumes, fish and wheat germ. [156] The majority of the lecithin is from soybeans; however, the use of egg extract lecithin is on the rise. Lecithin is a composition of the B vitamin Choline, linoleic acid and inositol. It has been documented that lecithin assists in not only lowering cholesterol, but also reducing cardiovascular disease. It also improves brain function and memory. It also aids in repairing a damaged liver from alcoholism, has shown promise in assisting in reducing complications due to AIDS, chronic fatigue syndrome, aging and rebuilding the immune system.

The protocol for lecithin is to take 1,200 mg 10 minutes before a meal. Use room temperature water when taking jell caps or you can use a tablespoon of granules and sprinkle them on your food. Another method is to take a tablespoon of the liquid Lecithin a day. I have had some clients take two tablespoon of the liquid at separate times during the day.

Protein, the Building Blocks of Life

"You are a miracle. Science, no matter how well designed and executed, can never come close to the astounding capabilities of the human body and mind."

Stephen Cherniske, M.S.
The Metabolic Plan

Proteins are comprised of chains of amino acids linked together, which are essential to life. The word protein is derived from the Greek word "protos" meaning "first". Proteins like carbohydrates are composed of carbon, hydrogen, and oxygen. Nitrogen is added to its composition to assist in the generation and repairing of tissues.

Protein is three-fourths dry weight of most body cells and is second in abundance to water. This makes up the basic chemical of blood, collagen, hair, tissue, nails, hormones, enzymes, infection-fighting antibodies, nerve chemicals, muscles, and skin. It is the primary building block that promotes and regenerates cells and tissues to sustain life. Children's growth and development depends on protein more than adults who need it more for regeneration of the cells and tissues. Pregnant and lactating mothers need more protein than men and non-pregnant women.

It is needed to maintain the body's ph balance and to regulate water balance in the blood serum for cellular stability. The protein chemical reaction is important in the immune system to create antibodies in order to fight bacterial, viral infections and unhealthy fungi. Without protein the body would have no structure or be able to move, stand, run, jump or think.

The difference between plant and animal protein is in the number and arrangement of individual amino acids. The construction of proteins in living creations such as humans, birds, fungi, yeast, bacteria, lizards, plants, etc consist of twenty amino acid, however, eight of them are essential and can not be produced by the body. These eight essential amino acids are what make a complete protein, so they have to be introduced to the body through food or supplementation. If there are less than eight essential amino acids, there is no protein. The remaining amino acids are not essential because the body manufactures them through the combinations of foods and other chemicals within the body. Amino acids have to maintain a certain balance with each other in order to construct a protein molecule and affect the DNA/RNA code. The universe is comprised of thousands of amino acids, however, we are just concerned with the eight essential amino acids, that make proteins.

Amino acids are the framework of proteins forming long chains consisting of helixes, spheres and branched structures. These amino acids are unique in their ability to make a protein because of their number, varieties, chain structures and their DNA encoding in the nucleus of each cell. Amino acids are bonded by peptides, which comes from the Greek word "peptos" meaning cooked.

When vegetables, fruits, grains or fresh foods are eaten, they go through the digestive process and are reduced into different amino acids or free acids. This enables them to be absorbed into the blood stream and circulated throughout the bodies billion of cells.

THE EIGHT ESSENTIAL AMINO ACIDS

<u>HISTIDINE:</u> Controls mucus pathogens. It is an important element in semen's ability to impregnate the ovum and fertility. It improves and induces good hearing.

Complementary elements:
    Vitamins: B-5 (pantothenic acid), C, B-3 (niacin), Vitamin E
    Minerals: Potassium, Bromine, Sodium, Chloride, Chromium, and Zinc

Deficiencies: All matters dealing with injuries to the nerves that control hearing; unable to distinguish words. Female reproductive imbalances (sterility, abortion, still birth, and premature birth).

Foods: Alfalfa sprouts, beets, carrots, celery, chicory, cucumbers, dandelion greens, endive, garlic, horseradish, sorrel, spinach (uncooked), turnips (roots and tops), apples, papaya, pineapple, and pomegranate,

ISOLEUCINE: Regenerate the hemoglobin (red blood cells). Aids in muscle function, and it affects the eyes, hypothalamus, kidney, lymph glands, thymus, and pineal gland. During childhood through adolescence it regulates the thymus. From adolescence to old age it governs the spleen and maintains metabolism.

Complementary elements:
Vitamins: A, B-3 (niacin), C. B complex, B-15, E, B-12
Minerals: Chrome, Zinc, Calcium, Selenium, Magnesium, and Sulfur

Deficiencies: Urine disorders, lack of muscle tone, blood disorders, flu and cold symptoms

Foods: Beans, coconut, legumes, nut (except the cashews, chestnuts, and peanut), olives, ripe papaya, and sunflower seeds

LEUCINE: Treatment of urine disorders (especially maple syrup urine disease—when the urine has a sweet smell), good to lower blood sugar level, it aids in skin and bone healing. Leucine polarizes the left (levorotatory) side of the body. It counter balances Isoleucine.

Complementary elements:
Vitamins: A, B-complex, B-2, B-12, Folic Acid
Mineral: Copper, Manganese, Calcium, and Selenium

Deficiencies: The inability to lose or gain weight, spasms in the colon, problems of the digestive tract, liver congestion, and kidney disorders

Foods: Beans, coconut, legumes, nut (except cashews, chestnuts, and peanut), olives, ripe papaya, and sunflower seeds

LYSINE: Aids the liver and gallbladder in fat metabolism. Converts calcium for bone growth as it maintains cartilage and connected tissue.

It is an immune system balancer and prevents degeneration of tissues and body cells. It is very important in female disorder of the corpus luteum mammary glands, ovaries, and pineal gland. Vitamin C regulates lysine converting for body absorption. It corrects the herpes simplex virus imbalance. L-Lysine inhibits dental decay. It is the binding element of this Co-enzymes Lipioic Acid, Biotin and Pyridoxal Phosphate.

Complementary elements:
    Vitamins: Niacin, PABA, B-complex, A, B-2, B-5, B-6, B-15, and E
    Minerals: Chromium, Zinc, Rubidium, Iodine, Sodium, and Calcium

Deficiencies: Chronic fatigue syndrome and tiredness are linked to a deficiency of L-Lysine, a loss of muscle integrity, hypoglycemia (blood sugar deficiency), antidote to allergy to Brewer's Yeast and Methionine; lysine is displaced by arginine.

Foods: The herbal food Comfrey is a rich source of lysine. Alfalfa, beets, carrots, celery, cucumbers, dandelion, parsley, soy beans (tofu), spinach (uncooked), turnips, apples, apricots, grapes, papaya, and pears

L-METHIONINE: Has a high concentration of the sulfur. It is part of the lipotropic team, including Choline and Inositol. Kidney and liver cell depend on this amino acid for regeneration. It also aids in the removal of waste and poisons from the liver. The serum and tissues benefit from this amino acid is important to the blood hemoglobin. L-Methionine maintains balances in the spleen, pancreas, and lymph glands. This amino acid prevents destruction of vital organs, tissues and necrosis. It hinders accumulations of excessive fat in the liver, as its production of lecithin increases, preventing cholesterol build up in the systems. Because of its high sulfur constitution, L-Methionine protects against cancer and slows down the aging process. At the same time it neutralizes free radicals and dispels toxins from the body. It synthesizes protein and is a fat allergy antidote. Hair growth is also stimulated by this amino acid.

Complementary elements:
   Vitamins: A, C, B-5, B-12
   Minerals: Chromium, and Zinc

Deficiencies:
   Loss of hair, poor skin quality, sore throat, enlargement of tonsils, cancer, high cholesterol, liver and gallbladder disorders, and body toxicity,

Foods:
   Brussels sprouts, cabbage, cauliflower (uncooked), chives, egg yolks, garlic, horseradish, onions, the herbal food sarsaparilla, watercress, apples, pineapple, Brazil nuts, and filbert nuts,

L-PHENYLALANINE: Aids the brain in the manufacturing of Norepinephrine, (neurotransmitter) which is a chemical that transports brain signals along nerve neurons to communicate with the body. The thyroid gland depends on this amino acid to secrete the hormone thyroxin, which is rich in iodine. It eliminates food, tissue, and cell waste from the body. It is valuable in learning and memory function as well as releasing all forms of depression (manic depression, schizophrenia, endogenous, and withdrawal syndrome). Phenylalanine suppresses the appetite as it increases energy levels, through releasing the hormone Cholecystokinin from the brain into the body systems. The kidneys and bladder balance rely on this amino acid.

Complementary elements:
   Vitamins: A, B-3, C, B-complex, B-15, E
   Minerals: Calcium, Selenium, Magnesium, and Sulfur

Deficiencies:
   Emotional imbalances, eye illness, depression, tumors, weight gain, appetite disorders, Thyroid imbalances, (NOTE: Administering too much Phenylalanine may result in headaches, irritability, and insomnia.)

Complementary elements:
   Minerals: calcium, selenium, magnesium sulfur
   Vitamins: A, B complex, B-3, B-15, C, and E

Glandular influences:
Eyes, hypothalamus, Pineal Gland, and Thyroid,

Foods:
Beet, carrot, cucumbers, parsley, spinach (uncooked), tomatoes, apples, and pineapple

L-THREONINE:
This amino acid is a catalyst between other amino acids and the body. Having a lipotropic action threonine prevents the liver from fat build-ups. The digestive and intestinal tract is aided in operating smoothly with this amino acid. It is one of the major amino acid with elastin, collagen and enamel proteins. It helps the uterus maintain its health and well-being.

Complementary Elements:
Vitamins: Folic Acid, B-Complex, B-12,
Minerals: Copper, Manganese, Calcium, and Selenium

Deficiencies:
Gastrointestinal problems, acid imbalance, fat allergies, sore throat, malnourishment and lack of assimilation, female disorders, painful and menstruation cycle difficulties (also known as dysmenorrahea), spotting, cysts on the ovaries, and fluid retention in the ovaries.

Elements of balance:
Minerals: calcium, copper, manganese, selenium
Vitamins: A, B complex especially B-2, 12, and Folic Acid

Glandular influences:
Appendix, lymph, skin, stomach, thymus, and tonsils

L-TRYPTOPHAN: It provides an efficient optic nervous system. This amino acid is useful in promoting good digestion, as well as aiding the body assimilate the B Vitamin Complex especially B6. Tryptophan is found in every cell of the body. When it is converted to serotonin (which reduces the brains electrical activity), Tryptophan acts as a neurotransmitter inhibitor and induces sleep. It also provides emotional stability and is useful for depression and stress related imbalances. Another quality of Tryptophan is its ability to elevate the histamine levels in blood, as well as stimulate growth hormones. It lowers cholesterol and fat in the blood system, as it regulates blood pressure through dilating blood vessels. The high level of Nicotinic Acid (Vitamin B-3 Niacin) in this amino acid counter balances cigarette smoking.

Deficiencies:
Nervous disorders, insomnia, joint dysfunction, poor skin tone, cigarette addiction, indigestion, schizophrenia, brittle fingernails, and arthritis.

Complementary elements:
Minerals: calcium, magnesium, selenium, sulfur
Vitamins: A, B-3 (Niacin), and E

Glandular influences:
Liver, lungs, lymph, parathyroid, spleen, and thymus

Foods:
Alfalfa, beets (whole plant), brussel sprouts (uncooked), carrots, celery, chives, dandelions greens, endive, fennel, spinach (uncooked), string beans (uncooked), and turnips (whole plant)

L-VALINE:
Valine is used in conjunction with Leucine, and Isoleucine to treat sugar in urine (Maple syrup urine dis-ease). These three amino acids have to balance each other in the body for optimum utilization. The body needs Valine for good muscle coordination. Valine is essential for female glands (ovaries, corpus luteum, and mammary glands). Aides the nervous system in elector impulse transmissions and it also helps in maintaining a sharp memory.

Deficiencies:
Nervous disorders, spitting up of blood, skin inflammation, biting fingernails, alcohol abuse, emotional and mental disorders, insomnia, throat and rectum inflammation.

Complementary elements:
 Minerals: copper, magnesium, manganese, sulfur,
 Vitamins: A, B complex, C, and E,

Foods:
 Almonds (raw, unbleached, unsalted), apples, beets (whole plant), carrots, celery, dandelion, lettuce, okra, parsley, parsnips, pomegranate, and squash (uncooked) tomatoes,

Therapeutic Strategy

"If nutrition were understood, and prevention and natural treatments were more accepted in medical community, we would not be pouring so many toxic, potentially lethal drugs into our bodies at the last stage of disease."

T. Collin Campbell, PhD and Thomas M. Campbell II

Studies show diabetes is a multi nutritional deficiency disorder due to mal-absorption, leading to malnutrition. The ability to correct and reverse diabetes is through nourishing cells, tissues, organs and systems of the body aiding the body in healing without pharmacology. Medical science provides medication to control the symptoms of diabetes without understanding the root cause leading to life long drug usage. Nutritional deficiencies have to be addressed in a manner where the body receives the proper nutrient over a period of time creating a balance within the digestive tract affecting the pancreas and other organs involved.

In order to facilitate this you have to take micronutrients (minerals and vitamins) and phytonutrients (herbs), change your eating habits and exercise on a consistent basis. On my protocol I have my clients take supplements for five days each week. The reason for this is to provide the body with nutrients and also allow it to work with the supplements in order for it to engage in it's own healing. When we use supplements or medication on a daily bases without a break the body does not have a chance to assist in it's own healing so the ailment continues to persist and grow to where the medication increases or the medication is changed to a stronger one. Many cases of side effects and toxicity from pharmaceuticals, herbs, minerals and vitamins are due to the consistent consumption without a break in between. This consistency does not allow for the body to detoxify the substance taken, so the body becomes overloaded and begins to work to eliminate the toxic material in the form of a side effect. The build up of toxic chemicals in the body places an extra burden on the body and it also interrupts the ability of the body to heal.

Supplements are just that, they are to assist the body in its ability to maintain life and health, they are not to take over the processes of the body, this is why they are called supplements. A person may take a multi-mineral/vitamin supplement, which may address their nutritional issue. However, in most cases when there are deficiencies a person has to take additional minerals and vitamin that may also be contained in the multi mineral because their body is in such a deficient state the body needs to exceed the Daily Recommended Value (RDA).

When the body is deficient in nutrients it is difficult to determine how deficient it is without lab analysis. The ideal protocol is to get a lab analysis and proceed from there; however it is not always possible to get a lab report that identifies nutritional deficiencies. Without the lab report there are several other methods of working to determine the nutritional needs. One of the other methods is Applied Kinesiology or Muscle Testing, which has worked well in establishing a person's nutritional needs. The other is from research where micronutrients have been identified as deficient is specific disparities.

We have to always remember the body is a chemistry factory and when the chemistry is correct it will function properly and when the chemistry is off there will be some health challenges. With this in mind the chemistry of the body is filled with minerals, vitamins and other nutritional elements, which need to be maintained for health.

We know the regeneration of cells, tissues and organs slow down with the aging process and the body is unable to receive nutrients in the same manner. The digestive tract gets slower decreasing the ability to absorb nutrients from food. The emotions constrict the growth and development of the cells, tissues and organs. Just being able to maintain a healthy body that does not have a lot of health challenges is a lot of work, so you know when there is diabetes it is three times more work to maintain health.

Supplementation of micronutrients and phytonutrients is extremely important in the ability to reverse diabetes. Without the assistance of supplemented nutrients diabetes will continue to exist for a lifetime.

The goal of this plan is to utilize micronutrients and phytonutrients to assist the body in restoring its ability to maintain health as it reduces and/or eliminates diabetes. It is to increase a person's nutritional value and improve their health and wellbeing. This is done through the use of nutritional supplementation and lifestyle changes.

Through the use of supplementation and lifestyle changes you will find your body dynamic change, an increase in the metabolic process, reduction of elevated blood glucose levels, lose weight and deceased high cholesterol levels. You will find energy levels improve, along with the elimination of specific food cravings (salt, sweets, etc) and the body will feel alive. The dosage of these nutrients has to be in such a proportion where they increase absorbability of nutrient in order to promote health. Each deficient nutrient has to be increased in away where you are able to see the affects of the nutrients in the reduction of your blood sugar levels and any other complications aligned with the diabetes. The protocol is to improve the uptake of glucose in a timely manner through using supplemented nutrients.

After sometime on the protocol you will find the dosage of the micronutrients and phytonutrients decrease as your blood sugar levels stabilize and your health improves. The key to reversing diabetes is to follow the protocol because over the years it has been shown to work very well for people with diabetes and its complications.

Protocol of Health Elements for Diabetes

"These are strange times, when we are healthier than ever but more anxious about our health"

Roy Porter
The Greatest Benefit To Mankind
A Medical History of Humanity

Even though, this book is about diabetes, it also address overweight and obesity, which are part and parcel of diabetes. The children are the future and many of them will have adult dis-eases before they are adults. By using the protocol I have laid out for you will find that your weight reduces as your health improves.

The protocol is not a diet, but a lifestyle change that should be with you for the rest of your life. You will also see where I use the word "eating habit" appose to the word "diet". When I think of a diet I always ask myself who is dying. Diets are normally temporary, for weight lose or a specific health condition. Humans like lower animals have the habit of eating nourishing foods to maintain health and well being and not dieting. To heal form weight or any other condition you have to change your lifestyle. When you change your lifestyle then you don't have to worry about the weight coming back or the health issue returning. Life style change is not as hard as you may think. The issues is you have been conditioned and it seems difficult to think about changing that conditioning. I had a lady who has another illness who said she really wanted to get well, but she would do anything but change her eating habits. I gave her information she needed and let her go on her way. Well, about six months later she called me asking me if there was something she could do about the condition because it got worse. I gave her the same suggestion I gave her the first time. Her reply was "I think I need to change my life." Another three months went by and she called me again, this time she sounded happy and full of joy. She was calling to let me know that she finally changed her lifestyle and it was as easy as I had told her it would be and her condition was getting better after all these years and all the many doctors she has encountered.

I am saying this to say that lifestyle change is not hard, it is about what you want for your health and sticking with it. The food changes you have to make along with exercise on a regular basis is worth it if you are able to increase your life by 5, 10, 15 years and live it without pain, suffering and a lot of medicine.

Here are a few tips, although I provide a protocol in the back of the book.

One of the first things you want to do is stop eating and drinking at the same time. It is an overwhelming cause of mal-absorption of nutrients by your cells.

Learn to chew your food and not gulp it down. Allow for it to become saturated with digestive juices in the mouth before swallowing. Overweight and obesity are directly related to gulped food.

Learn to combine your food well. This aids in proper digestion, absorption and assimilation, and elimination of waste byproducts in a timely manner.

Don't eat junk, fried, processed, overcooked or precooked food. They have been depleted of enzymes and furthermore they deplete the body's enzymes.

Find an exercise routine you like—one that fits your personality. Don't do the exercise just because it is the latest trend. Exercise should work for you and not against you.

Lastly do not eat when you are under stress or duress. It compromises your digestive tract.

Micronutrient

"A happy working of the human machine depends upon the harmonious activity of the various component parts. If all these work in an orderly manner, the machine runs smoothly. If even one of the essential parts is out of order, it comes to a stop."

Gandhi

The Wonders of Co Enzyme Q 10

Co Enzyme Q 10 also known as "ubiquinone" is an element that is a major part of the cell known as the mitochondria and is the energy producing element of the cell. It is a powerful antioxidant, immune stimulator, with anti aging properties, and reduces the prevalence of cardiovascular disease. When deficient it can cause cardiovascular disease, periodontal disease, and lack of energy, impaired immune functions, and even muscular dystrophy. Research shows it has been used to treat diabetes, obesity, Alzheimer's disease, candida, multiple sclerosis, balance heart rhythm, normalizes blood pressure and aids in reducing and/or eliminating elevated cholesterol with success. It aids in weight loss because of increased storage of brown fat. Research has indicated Q 10's ability to improve neurotransmission making it good for diabetics who have neuropathy. It has also been researched that CoQ10 can safely be taken up to 2,500 mg, however, for the best absorption it needs B complex and iron and the excessive sugar inhibits absorbability of CoQ10.

Depending on your situation I suggest you begin with 200 mg of with a meal, however, if there is any other complication (neuropathy, etc) then you should increase the doses to 400mg. if you have type 1 diabetes you should be taking 250-400mg a day. Use this dose until the blood sugar reduces and then reduce the dose to 100-150mg a day.

CoQ10   RDA: 200-600 mg

A Family that Stays Together Heals Together (Vitamin B Complex)

The B vitamins are a family of synergistic vitamins working efficiently in the body. Their work has to do with metabolizing starches, proteins, fats (lipids) and sugars. They are water soluble, meaning they do their work in your body and they are execrated through the kidneys as urine. When they are released the urine has a slight faint aroma with a neon color and there has been no information on any toxicity or side effects. They are easily lost during storage and cooking. B vitamins are destroyed by excessive amounts of sugar and alcohol and diabetic need an increase in B vitamins.

Vitamin B Complex 200 mg you can take a supplement as well as consuming foods high in B vitamins. B complex has the full range of B vitamins and it is required when taken any of the other B vitamins. Because it has the full range of the complex to assist in the absorbability of the other B vitamins.

Vitamin B_1 (Thiamine): aids in digestion, production of Hydrochloric Acid, improves bowel transit time, assist in the stimulation of the entire nervous system, eliminates depression, improves the gastrointestinal system, converts excessive carbohydrates into fats for storage in the adipose tissues.

RDA 1.0 mg (milligrams), up to 100 mg can be consumed therapeutically.

Requirements for absorption: magnesium, vitamin B complex, vitamins C,& E, manganese, and sulfur

Signs of Deficiencies: beriberi (disease causing severe lethargy, fatigue, and it affects the cardiovascular, nervous, muscular and gastrointestinal systems.), depression, constipation, lower extremity numbness.

Causes of Deficiencies: Refined carbohydrates, alcohol, teas with tannins, prescription drugs dilantin (there may be other pharmaceutical drugs that cause a deficiency of this vitamin.)

Sources: beans, Brewer's Yeast, blackstrap molasses, brown rice, eggs, fresh vegetables, meat (organ), nuts, whole grains, milk.

Vitamin B 2 (Riboflavin): aids in reducing cataracts, mouth infections and sore, split nails, skin imbalances, assist in the digestion and absorption of carbohydrates, fats, and proteins, aids in the formations of red blood cells, reduction of anemia, and balance of hormonal levels. It plays a role in neurotransmission and aid in reduction of depression.

RDA: males 1.5-1.7 mg females 1.3-1.2 mg pregnant women 1.6 mg lactating women 1.8 This vitamin has been consumed in dosages of 400 mg safely. It is recommended to administer 20 mg at a time for better absorption.

Requirements for absorption: B complex, vitamin C

Signs of deficiencies: burning lips, eruptions of the skin, indigestion, lethargy, loss of appetite, loss of vision, mental disorientation, oily hair, sores in mouth and tongue, split nails.

Causes of deficiencies: alcohol abuse, excessive amounts of refined sugar and carbohydrates, some prescription drugs like anti malarial drugs.

Sources: Brewers Yeast, Blackstrap Molasses, eggs, dark green vegetables, meat (organ), nut, rice polish, wheat germ, whole milk produces.

There has not been any record of side effects or danger of toxicity from this vitamin.

Vitamin B 3 (Niacin, nicotinic acid, niacinamide): aids in the release of energy from carbohydrates, proteins and fats, it assists in the formation of red blood cells, helps the body to detoxify from drugs and toxic chemicals, decreases elevated cholesterol, reduces the risk of heart disease, used in the treatment for pellagra and schizophrenia, improves the gastrointestinal system.

RDA: males 15-20 mg, females 13-15 mg, pregnant females 17 mg, lactating need more than 20 mg.

Requirements for absorption: B complex, vitamin C

Signs of deficiencies: indigestion, lethargy, loss of appetite, pellagra, schizophrenia, skin eruptions, weakness

Causes of deficiencies: alcohol abuse, excessive consumption of corn or cornmeal, use of tobacco products.

The side effects of niacin include skin flushing, and in time released capsules it has been related to liver damage. It has also been linked to gastric irritation, and nausea. The best and safest form is inositol hexaniacinate or Royal Jelly. Always take the B complex when consuming this vitamin.

Vitamin B5 (Pantothenic Acid), a hormone stimulator (Adrenalin, Cortisone), aid in reducing the affects of aging, hair loss, stress, an excellent vitamin for hypoglycemia, assists in the metabolic process of fat, carbohydrates, and proteins, promotes the development of red blood cells, has a significant ability to reduce cholesterol and triglycerides, it has been known to correct painful burning feet, is good for food allergies.

RDA 25-100mg there are no real daily recommendations for this vitamin do to the fact that deficiencies are rare and it can be found in many of the foods consumed.

Signs of Deficiencies: fatigue, burning painful feet, listlessness, numbness of the feet,

Sources: avocados, brewer's yeast, broccoli, brown rice, buckwheat flour, cashews, cauliflower, flour (rye, whole wheat), garbanzos, hazelnuts, kale, liver calf, lentils, mushrooms, peanuts (caution should be take when eating peanuts because of the afloatatoxins fungus), peppers (red chili), soybeans (soy products should be consumed in a fermented state for best digestion.) spilt peas, sunflower seeds, wheat germ (toasted), wild rice.

Folic Acid (folate, folacin, pteroylmonogluyamate): it is vital in cellular genetic coding of DNA, critical in fetal nervous system development, an essential element in normal growth, development and maintenance of the cellular structure, as a neurotransmitter it aids in regulating moods, sleep, appetite.

RDA: 400 micrograms (mcg)

Requirements for absorption: B12 (when teamed together they act as a methyl molecule (SAME). B6 with this vitamin combined with B12 the trio works to reduce homocysteine. Vitamin B complex, vitamin C

Signs of Deficiencies: all cells of the body are involved in this vitamin's deficiencies. Gastrointestinal disorders, reproduction system (spontaneous abortions, decreases infants death rate, abnormal pap smear, macrocytic anemia), poor growth in children, Neural Tube Defects, Atherosclerosis, depression, gingivitis, insomnia, loss of appetite, diarrhea, shortness of breath, canker sores, anemia, irritability, shortness of breath, forgetfulness.

Causes of Deficiencies: oral contraceptives, alcohol, sunlight, chemotherapy drugs, several types of pharmaceuticals,

Food Sources: apricots, asparagus, avocados, barley, beans, broccoli, cantaloupe, carrots, egg yolks, green beans, green leafy vegetables, meat (organ), milk, nuts, rye, wheat germ.

Vitamin B6 (Pyridoxine): assists in the metabolic process of converting fats, proteins, and carbohydrates into energy for the body to use. It has a special relationship with protein and its conversion to several different nutrients, like tryptophan to niacin. Pyridoxine has a wide variety of uses in formulation of red blood cells, nerve chemical stimulation like serotonin and functions to maintain emotional balance. Pyridoxine is essential in stimulating pituitary gland's function of cells potassium and sodium electrolytes balance. This vitamin is known for its ability to reduce and eliminate numbness of the extremities (neuropathy). The healing affect it has on the kidney can prevent kidney damage and failure, as we know many diabetics pass away from renal failure. In my therapy of diabetes I insist on clients taking Pyridoxine in a multi vitamin, B complex and an additional 250 mg, which over the years I have found helpful in eliminating any case of renal failure, and an increase in the ability to absorb nutrients. Because it is a water-soluble vitamin it does not accumulate in the body, it is seen in the urine.

RDA: 2.5 mg to 1,000 mg This vitamin has been known to be toxic at daily dosages of 2,000 mg or more for long periods of time. For best result maintain a daily dosage of 500 or below.

Requirements for absorption: B complex, Vitamin C, Magnesium, zinc, riboflavin, potassium and sodium

Signs of Deficiencies: anemia, lethargy, vomiting, dermatitis, depression, kidney stones, nausea, convulsions in infants, nervous system inflammation.

Causes of Deficiencies: alcohol, food dyes, pharmaceutical drugs including dopamine, hydralazine (used for hypertension), isoniazid (used in medicine for tuberculosis), and penicillamine (used to treat arthritis, kidney stones, lead poisoning, and skin conditions), oral contraceptive, and processed food.

Sources: avocados, bananas, blackstrap molasses, beans (cooked dried), beef (should be without medications), bran (wheat), brewers yeast, cabbage, cantaloupe, carrots, cauliflower, eggs (organic or free ranged), dried fruits (non sulfured), green leafy vegetables, green peppers (they are members of the nightshade family and can increase pain if you have joint pain), liver, nuts (peanuts and pecans), and wheat germ.

Vitamin B 12 (Cobalamin, Cyanocobalamin), is very instrumental in building and maintaining the cover around the nervous tissue (myelin sheath), aids in the replication of the genetic code of the cells (DNA), it is essential for the formation of neurotransmission, Vitamin B12 is a key element in regeneration and production of blood cells. It aids in the reduction of depression. Vitamin B 12 cannot be administered in the same method as other vitamins. It has to be administered either through an intravenous process or a sublingual process where you would place it under your tongue where it will be absorbed.

Signs of Deficiencies: anemia (pernicious), underdevelopment of the nervous system, numbness, tingling, mood swings, reduction in vision, dizziness, fatigue, poor cellular structure, poor blood clotting, bruising easily, and low blood pressure.

RDA 0.3-2.2 mgcs

Requirements for absorption: folic acid, vitamin B complex, vitamin C, calcium, choline, B 6, inositol

Causes of Deficiencies: Autoimmune disease, low levels of melatonin, malabsorption, increase in age.

Sources: bananas, bee pollen, Brewer's yeast, concord grapes, eggs, meat (organ), miso (soybean paste), raw wheat germ, sunflower seeds.

The Power of Vitamin C

Vitamin C is a water-soluble vitamin that is essential for health and well-being. Vitamin C can be found in fat soluble forms (Palmatate) as well, however, most of the vitamin C used is in either the form of ascorbic acid, Rose Hips, citrus, or acercola hips. Vitamin C is one of those vitamins the body is unable to manufacture; even through it has many functions in the body.

Vitamin C is well known for maintaining the integrity of the gums and preventing Scurvy (bleeding gums). It maintains collagen, which is all of the connective tissues (ends of bone, spinal disc, blood vessel walls, tendons, etc.) heals wounds, bleeding gums, enhances the immune system, throughout the body. Vitamin C will assist in reducing the Sorbitol and inhibit glycosylation of protein. It assists in wound healing.[157] Vitamin C makes a large contribution to the rebuilding and maintaining of the immune system. In his book Encyclopedia of Nutritional Supplements, Dr. Michael T. Murray, ND state "From a biochemical viewpoint, there is considerable evidence that vitamin C plays a vital role in many immune mechanisms."[158] As we know type 1 diabetes is linked to immune deficiencies and vitamin C has been shown deficient in diabetics type 1 and 2., which indicates vitamin C is a great asset to diabetics. It also is an antioxidant working to reduce and/or eliminating free radicals. As a matter of fact together with vitamin E and glutathione they defend against cell damage from free radicals. [159]

RDA: 30-95mgs Vitamin C can be taken up to 3,000 mgs without side effects. When vitamin C is consumed in excessive levels there will be loose stools. If this occurs then just reduce or discontinue vitamin C and bowels will turn to normal.

Requirements for absorption: Bioflavonoid, calcium, vitamin E, beta-carotene, glutathione, and selenium.

Signs of Deficiencies: scurvy, immune deficiencies, colds, coughs, diabetes, poor wound healing, extensive bruising, depression, low sperm count, and glycosylation.

Causes of Deficiencies: tobacco smoke, sugar,

Sources: Acerola, broccoli, Brussel sprouts, cabbage, cantaloupe, cauliflower, collard greens, elderberries, green peas, green peppers, green mint, greens turnips, kale, lemons, lime, orange, parsley, raspberries, rose hips, rutabaga, strawberries, watercress, and watermelon

The Workings of Vitamin E

Vitamin E is a fat-soluble vitamin with antioxidant properties that assists other fat vitamins from being oxidized in the body's oxygen. It is also the only fat soluble vitamin that does not build up in the body and spends a shorter period of time in the body. Of all the different types of vitamin E, d-Alpha-tocopherol is the most effective and absorbable. Vitamin E is very instrumental in strengthening the heart and other muscles along with its scar tissue healing ability and its retardation of the aging process. If you have any conditions where you are taking blood thinners then you do not want to take vitamin E because it is a blood thinner in its own right and has the ability to prevent and dissolve blood clots.[160]

In his book Encyclopedia of Nutritional Supplements, Michael Murray, N.D. show two major examples of the healing and preventive power of vitamin E. He states, "Vitamin E provides significant benefits in protecting against heart dis-ease and stroke. He went on to say "Confirmed antiantherosclerotic effects of vitamin E include an ability to reduce LDL cholesterol peroxidation with an improvement in plasma LDL breakdown; inhibition of excessive platelet aggregation; increase in HDL cholesterol levels; and increase fibrinolytic activity."[161] In another statement Dr. Murray discusses the fact that diabetics have an increased need for vitamin E because of their high levels of oxidative stress and it increases insulin's activity and reduces the risk of cardiovascular disease in diabetics.[162]

RDA 150mg (males), 120mg (female) Note: Women who are pregnant or lactating need more vitamin E.

Requirements for absorption: vitamin A, B complex,

Signs of Deficiencies: Vitamin E deficiencies are rare, however, there are some areas where there could be low levels of vitamin E. celiac disease, postgastrectomy syndrome, sickle cell disease hemodialysis (many diabetic graduate to dialysis), cyctic fibrosis, thalassemia, nerve damage, animia,

Absorption: Vitamin A, B-complex, Vitamin C, Manganese, Selenium. As a matter of fact vitamin C and selenium really aid the antioxidant properties of vitamin E to work well in the body.

Inhibitors:

Food Sources: Broccoli, Brussels Sprouts, eggs, leafy green vegetables, soybeans (fermented) vegetable oil (non-hydrogenated), wheat germ, whole grain cereals,

Super Foods

> In the large scheme of things, the miracle these food essences continually perform inside our cells, outside our awareness, are very tiny.
>
> *Jean Carper*

Chlorophyll

Chlorophyll is such a wonderful substance that I really don't know where to begin. It is the green color of the plants. That green pigment that we see in plants is through a process known as photosynthesis. Photosynhthesis is the uniting of the sun's energy of plants, algae and grasses that turns them green. Photosynthesis is a process that the body is unable to preform.

According to Dr. Banard Jensen in his book "The Healing Power of Chlorophyll from Plant Life" he states "When we take this green into our body, the results have been short of miraculous, for chlorophyll is an all-around food beneficial for tissue repair. Anyone who takes liquid chlorophyll is helping to neutralize some of the sprays and abnormal materials from artificial fertilizers that get in many of the foods we buy."

Chlorophyll nutrients in plants provide the body with all the nutrients needed to assist the body in maintaining health and overcoming disease. Chlorophyll maintains these nutrients in perfect balance. Chlorophyll is a powerful blood builder. When we look at the hemoglobin of the red blood cell and compare it to the chlorophyll molecule, we find the only difference between the two is the center atom of the iron molecule is iron and the center molecule of chollophyll is magnesium. This is why chlorophyll has been used to increase iron and cleanse the blood stream of heavy metals and other toxins.

Chlorophyll, not only provides nutrients, but also increases the oxygenation of the cells allowing the cells to heal, cleanse and reduce the level of disease. Chlorophyll also contains a high level of Gamma Linolenic Acid (GLA). Research shows that diabetics are deficient in both magnesium and GLA. I have observed that when I place diabetics on two tablespoons of chlorophyll a day that it not only improved their blood sugar, but it increased their energy levels and digestion.

There are several studies showing how powerful chlorophyll is when healing the body. In one study reported in Nutrition & Cancer, Dr. Chiu-Nan Lai and his colleagues at the Department of Biology, The University of Texas System Cancer Center, which is an affiliate of the M.D. Anderson Hospital & Tumor Institute in Houston, the chlorophyll in wheat grass was used in cancer research. What the team found was that liquid wheat grass would inhibit the mutagenic effect of cancer. In other words, it reduced the ability of the cells to develop into cancer. [163]

Chlorophyll is found in what are characterized as Supper Foods because of their ability to provide complete protein, mineral, trace elements, vitamins, carotenes, and other phytochemical with healing powers. These foods include Spirulina, Wheat Grass, Barely Grass, Chlorella, and other sea vegetables.

Wheat Grass

Wheatgrass is a rich green grass full of chlorophyll from wheat berries that you would find on the top of the miracle and supper food list. Its notoriety came about by Dr. Ann Wigmore, the founder of the Hippocrates Health Institute in Boston. It has blood-purifying prosperities, and is filled with the all of the nutrients the human body needs in order to maintain health and fight disease. Wheatgrass has a high concentration of super oxide dismutase (SOD) a powerful antioxidant that fights free radicals, which cause cancer.

Barley Grass

Barley Grass is similar to wheatgrass in its composition However, in experiments at the George Washington University School of Medicine in Washington, D.C., conducted by Allen L. Goldstein, Ph.D, Head of Biochemistry, and his colleagues examined the relationship between leukemia and Barley grass. What they found was that the Barley grass extract eradicated 30 to 50 percent of the leukemia. With that type of power, it cleanses the blood and increases the ability of the blood to maintain nutrients that provide a positive effect on diabetes.

Chlorella

Chlorella has all the B vitamins, protein, vitamin C, amino acids, vitamin E and other trace minerals to aid the body to maintain its ability to heal and reduce the risk of contracting diseases. It is known to be very high in RNA and DNA and has the ability to increase the proliferation of the cells as it cleanses the blood stream. Chlorella is a 2 billion year old single cell algae that grows in fresh water and is high in chlorophyll, and beta carotene. As a matter of fact, the word chlorella comes from the Greek word "chloros" meaning green and "ella" which means small.

Studies have show chlorella is used to treat a number of health disparities with great success. The Sun Chlorella "A" funded a clinical trial at the Virginia Commonwealth University in 1986, where Professor Randall Merchant, professor of Neurosurgery and Anatomy, studied the effects of chlorella on the immune system. The results of the study shows that chlorella not only boosted the immune system, but also reduces cancer, brain tumors, decreases hypertension, fibromyalgia, and ulcerative colitis. Since that trial, Professor Merchant has continued to study the effects on chlorella on other health disparities including diabetes. His 2008 study revealed chlorella is ability to make the body less sensitive to insulin. He stated, "It seems that chlorella turns on the genes that control the way insulin is normally used by the cells in the body. This research shows that chlorella could in theory help correct the problems of metabolic syndrome. It is not a magic bullet, but taking it is another preventive thing you can do, like exercise or watching your diet." [164]

Enzyme Therapy

> When a person is lacking in one or more of these primary digestive enzymes, the food category associated with that enzyme does not get digested properly and that person is said to be intolerant to that food.
>
> *Lita Lee, Lisa Turner, Burton Goldberg*

Enzymes are the life blood elements of the body, maintaining life. Without them life would not exsit. Our exsitence depends on the amount of enzymes and their ability to work in harmony within the body. If the body does not have the proper amount of a particular enzyme then it is unable to serve the body. Enzymes are protein based molecules that perform specific jobs in the body, which includes digestion, absorption, and eliminations. They repair the body after trauma, detoxify the systems, and processes neurological and mental activities. Science has identified more than 2,700 enzymes in the human body that play a vital role in the metabolic and digestive function of cells, tissues, hormones, blood, body fluids, fats, carbohydrates, sugars, minerals and vitamins. They are the workaholics that maintain the body's homeostasis.[xx]

We are provided with a certain amount of enzymes at birth and as we grow older and consume prepared foods we deplete our supply of enzymes. We are all running around talking about the aging process, well that process is depending on how we use enzymes and replenish them. Cooked, processed, and junk food, along with alcohol, and drugs deplete large quantities of enzymes from our systems reducing the body's ability to protect its self from common and chronic health aliments.[165] Enzymes are biological chemical agents with several types of names including life force energies, life energy, life principle, vitality, vital force, strength and nerve energy. In his book Unlocking the Secrets of Eating Right For Health, Vitality and Longevity Enzyme Nutrition The Food Enzyme Concept, Dr Edward Howell states in his introduction, "Without the life energy of enzymes we would be nothing more than a pile of lifeless chemical substance-vitamins, minerals, water, and

---

[xx] Homeostasis is the maintenance of relatively stable internal physiological conditions as body temperature or PH balance

protein." He continued by saying "they are what we call in metabolism, the body's labor force." [166]

In most health literature we find very little information about enzymes, it is almost as if they do not exist. Yet they are the real healing force of the body. Medical science and traditional health care, along with fitness experts have guided us toward high protein eating habits because proteins build the body. This is true, but they could not carry out that function without assistance from enzymes. For instance proteins degrade in the hydrochloric acid environment of the stomach by the enzyme pepsin (also found in papaya and pineapple). When pepsin is low in the body protein degradation is inhibited and the protein is moved into the small intestines where it accumulates and putrefies. As a result of this undigested protein in the small intestines your abdomen distends, bowels become sluggish with an offensive smell upon evacuation with the risk of waste contaminating your blood increasing prevalence for health disparities.

There are three types of enzymes working within the body, metabolic, digestive and food. Each set of enzymes have a specific job to carry out in the body. The metabolic enzyme maintains all body functions, including development of cells and their membranes, development of tissues and organs. Digestive enzymes on the other hand assists the body in digesting, absorbing and assimilating nutrients from food and beverages. Their main function is to nourish the body. Food enzymes are found in raw food and they assist in the beginning process of digestion reducing the strain on the body and digestive tract when food is introduced to the body. Because of enzymes sensitivity to heat they die when heated through cooking.

Enzymes are sensitive to heat and light. Enzymes decompose at a temperature of 118 degrees Fahrenheit. Most foods are cooked at about 250 to 400 degrees Fahrenheit. Food manufacturers process food well over 2,000 degrees Fahrenheit to reduce and/or eliminate the bacteria in food. At this point, there is no life given properties left in the food. All the nutrients and enzymes have been destroyed and the food is a burden on the body. When cooked foods are consumed, the body has to produce enough of its own enzymes to digest the food, which depletes the body's supply. This causes weight gain, bowel problems and other health disparities. In children it can impede their growth and development. According to Dr. Howell, "The habit of cooking our food and eating it processed with chemicals and the use of alcohol, drugs and junk food all draw out tremendous quantities of enzymes from our limited supply." He goes on to say "Frequent colds and fevers and exposure to extremes of temperature also deplete the supply. A body in such a weakened, enzyme-deficient state is a prime target for cancer, obesity, heart disease or other degenerative problems." He concluded with stating, "A lifetime of such abuse often ends in the tragedy of death at middle age."[167] This is why when consuming a cooked meal you should take digestive enzymes to assist the food in its process of digestion, absorption, assimilation and elimination.

The consumption of raw and fermented foods (sauerkraut, miso, tofu, etc, which are pre-digestible) provide their own enzymes, which assist in the digestive process. Eating raw or partially cooked food provides the body with a greater amount of enzymes, which improves ones nutritional values. Raw fruits and vegetables contain an abundance of enzymes that promotes and assists the body in maintaining health and well being. The enzymes in fruits and vegetables increase the body's chance of preventing and eliminating health conditions. Raw foods are also full of antioxidants, carotenes, phenols, carbohydrates, fats and sugars that work in harmony to increase health.

During dis-ease or exercise there is a greater demand for enzymes. If there is a deficiency the body tries to receive nutrients from wherever it can, leaving some areas of the body depleted. In the replenishing state, the body will shut itself down, resulting in fatigue; muscle cramps, and overall body weakness. This is when you may feel tired in the middle of the day or right after exercising.

The National Enzyme Commission identifies enzymes by the elements they act upon and place "ease" at the end of their name. For instance, protease synthesizes protein in the stomach, lipase breaks down fats in the small intestine; cellulase synthesizes cellulose in the small intestine, amylase breaks down starch in the mouth and maltase digests sugar in the small intestine. Some enzymes do not carry ease in their name like trypsin and pepsin degrades protein in the stomach.

Digestion and absorption relies on enzymes to break down food into liquids to be absorbed in the body. This is why it is important to chew (masticate) your food well. When we do not masticate our food well and it is swallowed in large pieces or eaten in the wrong combination, the "amylolytic" process of the alkaline environment of the mouth is unable to digest starch and carbohydrates. When proteins are consumed, which is a group of amino acids; they need protease a "proteolytic" enzyme to digest them in the acid environment of the stomach. If there is an enzyme deficiency, protein is unable to be digested. The protein moves into the small intestine where it putrefies and causes obstructions in the bowels. Without the absorption of protein, the body will have problems with growth and development.

Fats or lipids, which are triglycerides, phospholids, and sterols, need "lipolytic" enzymes to assist in the decomposition of its structure. In cases where fats are present but there is a lack of lipases to degrade them, they lodge in other areas of the body, such as in the blood as cholesterol, or in the adipose tissues as fat or cause other health issues.

As a diabetic you have to take digestive and metabolic enzymes on a daily basis with a meal in order to reduce and/or eliminate diabetes. Diabetes is a multi-digestive dis-ease and it has to be treated like one. After about a month or two you will see the difference in your blood sugar levels, bowels and energy.

Phytonutrients

"The highest form of ancient healing made no attempt to cure disease but rather sought to sustain the individual through the use of mild foods, herbs, and spiritual disciplines as the individual healed himself, from within and completely, body, mind and soul."

Michael Tierra, The Way of Herbs

Herbal Therapy

Natural plant life growing throughout the world are scientifically referred to as either herbs or phytonutrients with a variety of health and healing properties. These properties assist the body in its ability to maintain health. Herbal medicine is older than the human race, playing a vital role in many of the world's cultures. It has been passed down from generations to generations for health and healing. The history of Pharmacology (drug components) has identified phytonutrients as components of many pharmaceuticals (medical drugs). Herbs reinforce the body's essence, balances body fluids and tonify the organs to reverse several health disparities including diabetes.

A large amount of phytonutrient research is conducted in Germany, China, and India. Some of their research has been vital in reducing health disparities around the world. In many cases the human studies reflect the need to do more research, which expands the research of phytonutrients in other directions. The United State is very slow in their willingness to spend the monies in major phytonutrients research. There is some money spent, but not even close to the amount spent in other counties. The National Institute of Health (NIH) has a Complementary Alternative Medicine (CAM) division that looks at health disparities and the use of micronutrients, phytonutrients, massage, acupuncture, and other modalities that are not (western) traditional healing arts. This is the site of most of our research. Most other funding sources are afraid to spend money on CAM because it has not really been sanctioned by the American Medical Association. This is why many doctors will not honor the use of micronutrient and phytonutrients therapy for health disparities. However, the newer generations of doctors are being introduced to the world of CAM. Some of them are embracing CAM with open arms and others are not sure about using it in their practices.

Each phytonutrient in my protocol has been used and researched to identify their constituents, healing properties, dosage, and any toxic affect they have. In the literature on the phytonutrients I have found the best method of administering the phytonutrient, its time of day and in many cases it organ of choice. My formulations have been developed and used over the past 15 years with great success in assisting the body to rebalance it's self and work to reduce and/or eliminate diabetes, as you will see in the case studies presented later. I also include in my protocol several traditional Chinese herbal formulas that support my formulas in the ability to reduce and/or eliminate diabetes.

Di Gui Pi Ren Shen: This formulation is to reinforce, balance and tonify the nutritional and energtical values of the body where the blood cells begin to promote health and well being and they uptake glucose. The herbs in it have shown in research to provide the body with the needed nutrients so it can reduce elevated blood sugar levels.

Liu Wei Di Huang Wan: For centuries the Chinese herbal doctors have administered this formula to rebalance kidney yin (water-left kidney) and the liver (stored blood). This is one recommended for diabetes, chronic nephritis, optic nerve atrophy, and central retinitis.[168] It has also been used in treating renal failure.

You Gui Wan: This ancient Chinese formula is used to Restore the Right Kidney (Pill). It is the source pill to tonify the yang (active energy). It is used for weakness in the lower back, impotence, spermatorrhea, infertility, incontinence and edema. Many diabetics experience some or all of these deficiencies. It also assists in tonifying blood-creating circulation. When working with the kidneys it is best to tonify and balance both kidneys at the same time. [169]

Gui Pi Tang: In Traditional Chinese medicine the Spleen and Stomach major organs of digestion and have a vital role in diabetes. The spleen is one of the hardest working organs in body and most of the time it is deficient, impacting blood sugar levels. The spleen manufactures blood from the foods consumed and assists in it circulation throughout the body in Traditional Chinese Medicine. On the other, hand the stomach is the discriminative organ deciding where and how the food will enter the systems and is the major site of diabetes. Gui Pi Tang (Return the Spleen

Decoction) balances the Spleen allowing it to function in a manner that aid in regulating the uptake of glucose and influence the activity of the stomach. Gui Pi Tang is also known for its ability to reduce and/or eliminate numbness in the upper and lower extremities. [170]

Bowel Enhancer: as I stated 98.5 percent of type 2 diabetics are constipated, which can be seen in the distention of the abdomen where the small intestines are filled with waste and nutrients are not being absorbed. This formulation does not have any laxative properties. It is a fiber base product that reinforces peristalsis (wave in the colon) and absorbs toxic waste assisting in moving waste out of the body. Because of the elements within this product it also assists in the detoxification of the phase II of the liver, moving heavy metals and other toxins from the body.

Wood Detox: The liver plays an important role in diabetes and the maintenance of the entire body. It contributes over 100 different functions and is a primary detoxifying organ (phase I (water) and phase II (fat). It also stores blood, transposes glycogon to glycogen to glucose, where it has a devastating affect on blood sugar. When toxic it can influence blood in a negative manner creating several different imbalances such as numbness, tingling of the extremities, elevated blood pressure and/or cholesterol, etc. The combination of phytonutrients in Wood Detox align itself with the detoxifying process of the body and assists in the process as it also promotes nourishment. During this process the liver has the ability to detoxify itself in both phases and work to reduce and/or eliminate toxins from the body. The sour principle of some of the phytonutrients in this formulate increase the livers ability to manufacture bile, secrete it to the gallbladder where the gallbladder stores it before secretes it into the small intestines, which increases the small intestines ability to move toxic waste to the large intestine for expulsion. This formula has been used in our Detox program for the past 20 years with success in assisting the body in its process of detoxification.

Qing Xiang: in conjunction with diabetes many diabetics are overweight and have hypertension (high blood pressure). This formulation increases the body's nutritional values in order for the body to address hypertension. When the body has a balance between sodium and potassium, or a reduction in cholesterol the blood pressure is normal, however, when this balance is upset the blood pressure rises. Some of the phytonutrients of this formulation contain potassium and work with the body to increase its' potassium levels, which reduces blood pressure. This formulation works well with the above formulas to aid the body in its ability to heal.

The formulas are the major ones I recommend to my clients that we produce. There are other formulas and phytonutrients that have been researched to reduce elevated blood glucose levels. I will identify some of these herbs.

Bitter Melon (momordica charantia)

Bitter Melon has been known throughout the world for its ability to decrease blood sugar levels and improve glucose tolerance. It has been noted that in one case study, Bitter Melon may be responsible for the renewal and recovery of the pancreas insulin producing Beta cells.

Bilberry (Vaccinium myrtillus)

Bilberry reduces high blood glucose levels in type 2 diabetes with success. Many people know Bilberry for its eye health properties, however, it is becoming known for the anthocyanosides. Bilberry is a blood sugar reducer that is not as strong as insulin, but benefits diabetics and many complications associated with diabetes.

Fenugreek (Trigonella foenum-graecum)

India has conducted clinical trails using large doses (25 grams) of Fenugreek to reduce high blood glucose levels. [171] It contains the amino acid hydroxyisoleucine, that stimulates the pancreas causing it to secrete insulin. Its interaction on the intestinal tract allows a slow release of glucose into the blood stream enhancing the bloods ability break down the glucose and absorb it into the body after a meal.

Gymnema sylvestre (Gurmar meshasringi cherukurinja)

This Ayurvedic herb stimulates the pancreas to manufacture more insulin as it reduces high blood glucose levels. It inhibits the taste of sugar on the tongue.

Acid/Alkaline-Ph balance

"Minerals, vitamins, proteins, chlorophyll and enzymes are the keys to health. Together, they maintain our cells and work to correct any abnormal condition that occurs."

Yoshihide Haiwara, M.D.

We eat food for fuel, energy, and to nourish our body. When foods are eaten in the right combinations, chewed well without drinking at the same time, they don't putrefy or ferment in the small intestines. On the other hand, when there is a disruption in the process of eating, then foods are able to putrefy or ferment in the body creating waste deposits in the small intestines. The whole purpose of eating is to nourish our cells, which develop into tissue, producing organs, promoting healthy body systems and creating a neutral acid/alkiline balance. This acid/alkiline balance is universal and is known as Ph

Ph means Hydrogen Potential ions. Without going into great detail about Ph, I will simple say Ph balance is the level of oxygen cells receive in their process of regeneration and promoting health. The importance of Ph is in the amount of oxygen cells receive. The human body's Ph should be from 7.35 to 7.45. When it is in that range cells oxygen level are alkiline promoting good health. If for any reason Ph decreases, even by a fraction of a point the cell's begin to lack oxygen, become acidic and promote dis-ease. Every living organium and none living enites has an acid/alkline balances determining the balance of their existence.

Ph balance is calculated in a range of numbers that extent from 1 to 14 with 7 being at the neutral level and 1 through 6.9 being acidic and 7.1 through 14 being alkaline. Just as the body can be too acidic it can also be too alkaline and in a dis-ease state. It is good to work to maintain a close 7.35 to 7.45 as possible. When there is a good Ph balance the body will be healthy because the cells are receiving an abundance of oxygen promoting health.

Acidosis as it is referred to when the body is too acidic resulting in health disparities as insomnia, arthritis, water retention, abnormally low blood pressure, halitosis (bad breath), teeth sensitivity to vinegar and acidic fruits, foul smelling stools, migraine headaches, asthma, constipation, frequent sighing, bronchitis, stomach ulcers, malnutrition, obesity, diabetes mellitus, cancer, and many other health disparities. *Alkalosis* occurs when the body has too much alkaline and causes hyperventilation, night coughing, bone and heel spurs, gastric and peptic ulcer (from alkaline drugs), burning and itching sensation, dry stools, seizures, night cramps, hypertension, cracking joints, protruding eyes, nervousness, blood clots, and many other health disparities. It is best to try and eat foods that stabilize the body's PH balance at 7.0.

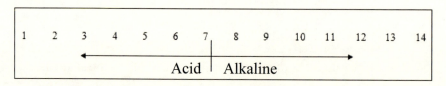

Foods and pure fresh water are naturally acid/alkaline balanced by nature and their balance changes when manipulated in food processing or in the body. When food is processed the chemical balance changes and has an effect on the body. This effect could be either acidic or alkaline depending on the food and the manipulation process. We have been taught that an orange is an acidic fruit, well when you eat an orange it becomes alkaline in your body, increasing oxygen to the cells promoting health.

This delicate acid/alkaline balance reacts to everything we ingest or wear for that matter. Women notice this more than men when they purchase earring that are not gold or silver. The earrings turn their ears green causing an infection, which is part of the acid/alkaline balance. The body's reaction to food or clothing is calculated in its ability to assimilate the substance and use its nutrients or cause a reaction of rejection gives an appearance of an allergic reaction. In this case, food substance reactions are because the body is over loaded with acidic waste reducing the elimination systems of bowel and kidney's capacity to expel waste. The waste either accumulates in the cells or it makes its way out of the body through the skin and sinuses where we refer to it as an allergy.

One of the issues in this society is we consume too many damp (acidic) foods. These foods are the causes of our health issues, robbing the body of its oxygen. It is a fact, when we consume more alkaline foods our health improves. This is the basis for the five fruits and vegetables a day. These foods, especially when consumed fresh and ripe are alkaline, full of enzymes, nutrients and oxygen to reduce the acidity that causes waste build up resulting in illness. Studies have shown germs are unable to live in an alkaline environment. Vitamin C is a good example of this when it is used for a common cold.

Alkaline foods and beverages have a powerful impact on the body, but when in excess, which is rare, they cause unhealthy conditions. This is why it is important for proper acid/alkaline balance. With in this chapter, you will find foods that are both acid and alkaline. You have to always remember "Its all about chemistry".

Acidic Foods

Dairy products (milk, cheeses, butter, ice cream), candy, cakes, soda, meats, fish, eggs, most beans, and peas, peanuts, many oils, canned foods, foods with pesticides, additives, and preservatives.

Alkaline Foods

Ripe fruits (dates, figs, apples, pears, melons, peaches, etc.), vegetables (carrots, parsnips, corn, broccoli, cucumbers, radishes, etc.), and whole grains such as millet, buckwheat, spouted legumes, barley, cracked wheat, brown rice, etc.

Combining Foods

"When essential nutrients are missing or unavailable your body is forced to function with hampered cells. Often this leads to extensive cell damage, causing cancer, disease, aging, and death."

Kim O Neill, Ph.D, Byron Murray, Ph.D
Power of Plants

It is interesting, humans are the most intelligent species of animal on the planet and have no clue about how to eat. All other aniamls have an instinctive approach to eating. They know when to eat protiens and how to separate the starches from the proteins as well as the proper combinations of food. Vegetarian animals naturally understand nutritional source of food to provide them with nutrients to maintain health and wellness. Carnivorous animals understand what meat to eat and which meats to leave alone. For instance, most carnoverous animals eat the organs and leave the carcus to rot. The vegetarian animals discriminate between starches and proteins. Each group of animals eat for health and not pleasure that is why they never have diabetes, hypertension, obesity or other health disparities.

Humans have never understood eating, the majority of us eat for pleasure and not for health, consuming any type of food, at any time of day or night in any combination and later finding our self with gas, constipation and ill health. The majority of us have no idea of how food is processed in the body and the chemical reactions taking places as we consume food. Once you have an understanding of the relationship between the chemistry of food then you may decide to combine your foods well or look at a different approach.

Keep in mind starch is digested in the mouth by the enzyme amylase, protein is digested in the stomach by the enzyme protease and the pancreas secretes the enzyme sucrose and maltase to digest sugar and lipase to digest fats in the small intestine. When the body becomes confused by improper combinations the body is unable to digest foods and store them in the small intestines as waste (for more on this subject read digestion on page 41).

The combination of food in each season assist in their proper digestion, assimaltion, and proper acid/alkaline balance. In the Spring consume 60% alkaline and 40% acid, during the Summer 50% alkaline and 50% acid. In the Fall and Winter, which are the cooler seasons you should consume 80-85% alkaline and 15-20% acid. This combination will increase the immune system and ward off any coughs, colds, or flus.

Eating foods in their proper combination is important for correct digestion, assimilation, and elimination of nutrients and food waste by products. When food is consumed in its proper combination, it harmonizes the organ network building the cells, tissues and organs improving the body's ability to stay healthy and creating longevity.

Food combining aids in balancing the energy force of foods in such cases where one food is missing an element and another one with that element is introduced to complete the element, like in the case of beans and grains. Grains are missing L Lysin, where beans have lysin but are missing L Mithinine. When combining them together they create a complete protein. However, when combining a protein with a starch it can cause fermentation in the intestines because starch is digested in the mouth and protien in the stomach. However, This is the result when the body has difficulty deciding which food should it digest first. Most vergetarians who don't eat any type of meat are deficient in protein and can use the combination of beans and grains.

Fruits

Fruits are cooling, cleansing, and alkaline food and for the most part they should not be cooked because heating them inhibits their enzymatic process reducing their cooling ability. They digest easy with little preparation times, however, there are some fruits like prunes whose properties are increased when heated. Because of their fibrous nature, many fruits stimulate bowel activity. A few things to remember about fruits.

Unripe fruits are acid-forming and do not properly digest in the intestinal tract, resulting in fermentation. Fermentation can cause bloating, gas, indigestion, toxic waste materials to be deposited in the blood resulting in other minor or major health conditions. Some dried fruits are acid-forming until they are soaked in water then they become alkaline and easily digested.

Here are some things to remember about fruits:

(1) Fruits are eaten separately from vegetables. Together they make a bad combination because fruits can take 60 to 90 minutes and vegetables can take 3 hours for digestion. The other thing is because of the fruit sugar it will ferment in the small intestine where it could develop into yeast.
(2) They are eaten in groups. Fruits should be eaten in groups like sweet with sweet, critics with critics, etc. When they are mixed their ability to digest could be inhibited. One reason is the mixture of acid with the alkaline consistency of sweet fruit can over burden the sweet fruit causing it to sit in the intestines and ferment.
(3) Never eat acidic fruits with sweet fruits
(4) Melons are always eaten by themselves. They digest quick and if inhibited they will ferment in the intestines. This is the best way to receive all of the nutrients from melons. Also they are foods with high water content allowing them to aid the urinary system and the fiber impact the bowels increasing both bowel movements and urination.
(5) Bananas are only eaten when they have little brown (freckle like spots). When bananas are eaten in their starch state that can ferment in the body aiding in the development of intestinal gas. The brown freckle like spots on their skin indicate they have changed from starch to sugar. There is a word of caution here for diabetics, which is you should stay clear of any form of banana because they will raise your blood sugar rapidly. In the case you do eat a banana, make sure you monitor you blood sugar level. They are good for diabetics when their blood sugar levels are low.

(6) Fruits should always be eaten ripe. Many of the fruits we eat are picked in mature and are acidic. The other thing is when eaten immature fruits will ferment in the intestinal system making way for yeast.

(7) Never put additional sugars of any kind on furit. Just think about it, if fruit has it's own sweet taste, then why would you need to add more sugar? If you have to add sugar to fruit then it is not ripe or it is over ripe. When fruit is over ripe you can taste it and even sugar wont improve the taste.

(8) Dairy products should never be consumed with fruits they are a protein fat. Pasturerized dairy products are acidic and mucous forming and when combined with fruit will not allow fruit to properly digest resulting in fermentation and putrefaction in the intestines creating congestion and other unhealthy conditions.

(9) Fruits and proteins are bad combinations. Again reducing the ability of the fruit to digest causing fermentation.

(10) Fruits and fats are bad combinations.

(11) Fruits and vegetables are bad combinations

(12) Fruits should be eaten by themselves and combine well with each other.

Fruits are filled with natural sugars and when allowed to sit in intestines for a period of time ferments and develops into yeast. This yeast can increase and leak through the small intestines into the blood turning to fat deposits, cholesterol, or yeast in the form of candida albercans an autoimmune disease, which is very difficult to rid from the body and requires a very special eating habit. This is one of the reasons you should not eat fruits with anything but fruits that combine well together and as a diabetic limited amounts of fruits.

Sweet Fruits						
Fresh Apircots	Banana	Carob	Dates		Dry Fruit	Figs
Melons	Pears	Persimmon	Pineapple		Prune	Raisins
Acerola Cherry	Apple(sour)	Cranberry	Currants		Gooseberries	Grapefruit
Grapes	Kumquats	Lemon	Loganberries		Oranges	Pineapple
Plums (sour)	Pomegranate	Tangerine	Tomatoes (eat separate)			
Sweet Fruits should be eaten by their self or as a group.						

Acid Fruits				
Apple	Avocados	Berries	Cherries	Grapes
Mangoes	Nectarine	Papaya	Plums	Raspberries
Acid fruits should be eaten by their self.				

Vegetables

Most vegetables combine well with proteins and starches. They are not good combinations with sweet foods or fruits. When combinated with these foods the fruits will ferment in the intestinal tract resulting in bloating, gas, waste gain and other internal conditions.

Vegetable are found in three different catagories, non-starch, mild-starch and starch. As a diabetic, it is best if you eat non-starch and mild starch vegetables, they will not increase blood sugar levels rapidly and they are easy on your digestive system. With them being easy on your digestive system you will be able to use the fiber from them to assist in promoting bowel movements.

Non-Starch Vegetables				
Asparagus	Bamboo Sprout	Bell Pepper	Beet (top)	Broccoli
Brussels	Sprouts	Cabbage	Cauliflower	Celery
Chard (Swish)	Chicory	Collards	Cowslip	Cucumber
Dandelion	Eggplant	Endive	Garlic	Green Beans
Kale	Leeks	Lettuce	Mushrooms	Mustard
Onion	Parsley	Peas (Fresh)	Radishes	Scallions
Sorrel	Spinach	Spouts	Swiss Chard	Turnip(Tops)
Zucchini				

Mild Starch Vegetables					
Beets	Carrots	Cauliflower	Parsnips	Rutabaga	Turnips

All cereals	Artichokes	Beans	Bread	Cauliflower	Cereals (Grains)
Chestnut	Corn	Crackers	Pasta	Peanuts	Potatoes
Pumpkin	Squash				

Starches

Starches should not be eaten with proteins, fruits, sugars, acid, fatty foods or dairy products. Starches are sugars and the ferment in the intestinal tract when they are combined improperly. Starches can be eaten with vegetables. As a diabetic you can eat some starches in moderation as long as they are whole grains. However, remember starch will increase your blood sugar levels. The difference in whole grain is that they will not increase your blood sugar levels very high and the levels will reduce quicker then refind starches. After eating any type of starch monitor your blood sugar to make sure you know where the levels are.

All cereals	Artichokes	Beans	Bread	Cauliflower
Cereals (Grains)	Chestnut	Corn	Crackers	Pasta
Peanuts	Potatoes	Pumpkin	Squash	

Fats

Fats are lipids that are digested by lipase an enzyme that breaks down fat molcues. Fats do not mix well with other foods. It makes it difficult for the lipids to digest when in the company of other foods, resulting in the accumalation of fat in the blood stream. This allows the fat to store in the adipose tissues causing weight gain and other health disparities.

All oils	Avocados	Butter	Cheese	Cream
Corn Oil	Cotton seed oil	Fat meats	Kefir	Lard
Margarine	Milk	Most nuts	Nut oil	Olives
Sesame seed oil	Sour Cream			

Fats/Protein

There are some foods that are both proteins and fats. These foods should be eaten by themselves.

Milk	Sour cream	Yogurt

Protein

Protein is the building block of all live creations and is needed to maintian the structure, tissues, and cells. Proteins should not be eaten with other foods because they will putrify in the intestines resulting in bloating, foul smelling gas, indigestion and other health disparitites.

Beef	Chicken	Eggs	Lamb
(all) Meats	Poultry	Pork	Sea Food

Protein/Starches

There are a variety of foods that are classified as both proteins and starchs that the body recognizes them as such and properly digest them. However, when you eat them with protein or starch they do not digest properly resulting in some type of gastoinstestinal disorder.

Dry Beans	Dry Peas	Millet

Sweets

As a diabetic, you should avoid or eat these foods with caution because they will increase your blood sugar levels very high. The only sweet you can safely use with out it increasing your blood sugar is Stavia. Sweets consist of any food or synthic substance provides a sweet taste or is constructed out of some type of sugar (sucrose, dextoses, maltose etc). Starch also brakes down into complex sugars, however, they are digested in the mouth instead of the small intestine. Sugars like starches should not be eaten with other foods because they will ferment in the intestinal tract resulting in toxins leaching into the blood and stored in the adipose tissues causing weight (waste) gain, or other health disparitites.

All Sugars	Acesulfame K	Aspartame	Barely Malt
Beet Sugar	Brown Rice Syrup	Brown Sugar	Confectioner's Sugar
Corn syrup	Corn sweetener	Cyclamates	Date Sugar Dextors
Fructose or levulose		Fruit Fruit Juice	Honey
Invert Sugar	Maple Syrup	Molasses	Raw Sugar
Saccharin	Sucrose	Turbinado	

Foods to Avoid

"The cornucopia of the American supermarket has thrown us back on a bewildering food landscape where we once again have to worry that some of those tasty-looking morsels might kill us."

Michael Pollan
The Omnivore's Dilemma

There are many foods a diabetic should avoid because they can increase blood sugar levels or they will not digest in the system and become trapped in the intestinal system where the waste will accumulate into the leaky gut syndrome. Some of the foods like dairy products will elevate cholesterol or increase the prevalence of type 1 or 2 diabetes. If a diabetic chooses to consume these foods they should have them in small portions and not very often.

Dairy products should be eliminated because they are linked to diseases like cancer, diabetes, high cholesterol, congestive heart failure, etc. This includes pasteurized milk, ice cream, cheese, which contains sulfates a cancer causing agent. If you are an African America, Jewish American, or Hispanic, you are more likely to be lactose intolerant. In the case you are a member of one of these groups of people, you should take a digestive enzyme when consuming these foods to assist in digestion and absorption of dairy products. Keep in mind that the research shows cow's milk is directly linked to type I diabetes mellitus (The Finland Study).

Sugar is a natural substance of the body in the form of glucose. Without it the body is sluggish and fatigue sets in along with the craving for sugar or sweets to increase blood sugar levels and create energy. However, when refined the nutrient in sugar cane is extracted and the sugar becomes empty calories that only increase the blood sugar levels and promote weight gain, but contributes to many of the diseases we are presently witnessing. Refined sugar also strips the body of B vitamins and other valuable nutrients. Sugar's are identified by many different names like barley malt, beet sugar, black strap molasses, brown sugar, cane pure sugar, carmel, corn syrup, date sugar, demeara sugar, dextrin, dextrose, fructose (high corn syrup), fructose (fruit), glucose, grape sugar, honey, inverted sugar, lactose, maltose, minitol, ample syrup, molasses, polydextrose, sugar (raw), sorbitol, sorghum, sucanat, sucrose, and turbinado. In the United States sugar of some form is in everything we eat, drink and it is even in smoking tobacco. This is one of the reasons we are so sick, because we are receiving empty calories in the form of sugar and no nutrients to nourish the body.

White flour products are a real minus to diabetics because it rapidly increases the blood sugar levels and having no nutrients to assist the body in its healing process. The bran from the wheat is stripped where all the nutrients such as B vitamins, chromium, and other vital elements are lost. The stripping of these elements makes white flour products difficult to digest resulting in several different types of health conditions. As a matter of fact, the government makes (manufacturers) synthetically replace some of the nutrients so there is value to consuming these products. This is the enriching process where manufacturer replace B vitamins, iron, thiamine, riboflavin, and niacin. When the nutrients are stripped from bran, it leaves a substance known as alloxan, which is known to cause diabetes.[172]

Hydrogenated (heated) oils are damaging to the body, tissues and cells. These oils increase the risk of atherosclerosis, cholesterol, obesity and diabetes. The heating process creating hydrogenation of cooking oils, have been known to leave amounts of aluminum and nickel in the body contributing to Alzheimer's disease. [173]

Alcohol ferments in the body turning to sugar. It has an ability to cross the blood brain barrier and influence the activity of the liver, resulting in emotional disturbances including anger, rage, forgetfulness, mental confusion unclear judgment and in some case death. Alcohol disrupts the ability of the cells to function normally. Alcohol has the ability to elevate blood sugar levels because the alcohol is a toxin and the liver works to clear the toxins from the body before promoting glucose into the blood stream. This is especially true in cases where alcohol is consumed without food being in the system.[174]

Eliminate any foods that are precooked, prepackaged, canned, boxed, or frozen. These foods have been overcooked, processed and have little or no nutrients. At a temperature of 118 degrees Fahrenheit the enzymes in the food die and have no life giving properties. They are also laced with chemical additives, preservatives, hormones, and other chemical that are not a component of the blood stream. This increases the prevalence of adverse health conditions.

Commercial teas, coffee, pasteurized sweetened juices or any drink labeled fruit drink are also harmful.

Healing Foods for Diabetes

"It is not enough to define health as the absence of disease. Rather, health is the aggregate of a series of specific conditions. These are ideal conditions and can in some way also be viewed as goals to be attained."

Annemarie Colbin

Apples (Malus domestica)

This ancient food is powerful in its ability to move the bowels and regulate the slow flow of sugar into the blood stream making it good for diabetics. It is known for its ability to promote digestion, which is something that is an issue with diabetics. Apples are high in vitamin A, C and calcium. The natural minerals and vitamins in an apple decrease high blood pressure and cleanse the blood vessels lowering the prevalence of hardening of the arteries, as well as purifying the lymphatic system. Apples are at the bottom of the glycemic index where their sugar to blood ratio is low but their power for healing is high. They are also a good food for diabetics to consume where the levels of their sugar has dropped. Because of the caffeine or chlorogenic acid in apples they have been shown to block the formation of cancer. [175]

Avocados (Persea Americana)

This food is a fruit that is full of calories and has 30 percent more fatty acids than any other fruit, however, Avocados is a monounsaturated fatty acid in the olelic acid family (same family as olive oil). Avocados are also high in fiber and provide an abundance of foliate and potassium making it good for people with diabetes, heart disease, high blood pressure. It lowers triglycerides and low density liproteins (bad cholesterol). The oils in Avocados have a negative affect on the drug "Warfarin" (Coumadin) a blood thinning drug. Avocados reduce the ability of this drug, making it less effective, however, when people stop eating avocados the drug works properly.

Beans (Legiminosae)

Beans are a staple of life. They are high in protein, low in fat, very high in fiber and consist of multitudes of minerals and vitamins. Their impact on the body wards off some of the negative effects of radiation and studies have shown they protect against cancer.[176] Beans have profound impact on diabetes and the ability to lower cholesterol. They are an excellent source of fiber and as a complex carbohydrate they release their energy slower so the body is able to absorb the nutrients and not elevate the blood sugar level. This aids insulin receptor sites in assisting cells to uptake more glucose out of the blood stream.

Buckwheat (Polygonaceae fagopyrum)

The Ph balance of buckwheat is neutral and has many different benefits to assist in the balancing of the body from lowering cholesterol to stopping cancer before it begins. It has a host of powerful nutrients like rutin, flavonoids, quercetin, magnesium, manganese, copper, zinc and has a very high quality of protein. Buckwheat is a good food for diabetes because its amylose and amyloprotein digests in a manner where its carbohydrates slowly enter the blood stream given the cells even distribution and a chance to absorb the sugar.

Bulgur

This is another fibrous food having amazing health benefits especially to those with cancer and diabetes. It contains Ferulic acid that reduces the risk of cancer from nitesamines which is derived from nitrates found in vegetable and nitrites that are components of cured fish, poultry, and meat and are cancer causing agents. Bulgur is a grain that also has the ability to reduce cholesterol decreasing the prevalence of heart attacks. Being fibrous it increases the movement of the bowels, slowing the increase of carbohydrates in the blood, aiding the cells in an even uptake of sugar into the cells reducing high blood sugar levels. As stated the majority of type 2 diabetics are overweight and their bowels are sluggish or they suffer with constipation. Bulgur promotes the release of this back up and sluggishness of the bowels, also reducing the risk of colon cancer and other bowel diseases.

Garlic (Allium staivum, niggrum)

Over the centuries garlic has been known as a miracle food because of all of the wonderful health benefits it provides. It is high in zinc making it vital for people with diabetes because many of them are deficient in this element. Garlic's concentration of vitamin C aids in the promotion of even uptake of sugar from the blood, which is a powerful diabetic treatment. Its high levels of zinc enable it to assist the insulin in the body to maintain a slow even level.

Onions (Allium cepa)

Onions are a sulfur based food that is the cousin to garlic and has many benefits to not just diabetes, also to hypertension as an antibiotic of which diabetics need during time of leg or other wound that need healing. Onions ability to lower elevated blood sugar levels has to do with the compound diphenylamine, which has the same affect as the drug tolbutamide used for diabetes according to recent Egyptian research. Diabetics also benefit from onions ability to lower cholesterol and blood pressure.

Parsnips (Pastinaca sativa)

It is a food that has both insoluble and soluble fiber blocking the intestines from fat and cholesterol absorption on one hand and on the other reducing the risk of cancer by diluting bile acids and increasing the movements of stools through the intestine. This makes Parsnips extremely good for diabetics because its insoluble fiber reduces the amount of its carbohydrates released in the blood stream at one time.

Spirulina (Arthrospira platensis)

This sea microalgae is filled with many types of nutrients to assist in building cells, tissues, and organs. It is powdered by the sun and chlorophyll that have a devastating healing affect on the body. Its components include gamma-linolenic acid (GLA) and arachidonic acid which are fatty acids the body needs for prostaglandins. The concentration of DNA and RNA is manufactured in its pigment and transferred in the consumption increasing the body's ability to improve its immunity and maintain health. Spirulina is known for its ability to lower cholesterol, improve the uptake of glucose, and assist in the reduction of weight. The effectiveness of Spirulina has shown itself in research of increasing the survival rate of mice with liver cancer.[177] Spirulina extract inhibits HIV replication in human T Cell peripheral blood mononuclear cells (PBMC), and Langerhans cells.[178]

At the 1974 United Nations World Food Conference, Spirulina was deemed the "best food for the future. During the conference the United Nation developed an intergovernmental organization for the Uses of Micro-algae Spirulina against Malnutrition. Their mission is to use Spirulina as a key element around the world to eradicate malnutrition.[179]

Diabetic Eating Plan

"As human beings, we originated from food, and food continues to sustain us throughout our lives. Ancestral and parental influences, especially the mother's way of eating, creates our physical and mental constitution. What we call heredity or genetic influence is simply the accumulated dietary and environmental influences of our parents, grandparents and ancestors."

Michio Kushi and Alex Jack
The Microbiotic Path To Total Health

As you engage in changing to a healthier lifestyle, you will need to think about meal planning. I don't provide recipes because there are a lot of them out there. However, I suggest you find some you like and modify them to fit your new lifestyle. The questions I am asked by my clients are, "What do I eat for breakfast and what is the biggest meal of the day? After you have taken all of the foods I like out of my diet, what is there left for me to eat?" Those are some of the questions I have had to answer over the years.

It has been said that breakfast is the most important meal of the day. You should understand that breakfast is Breaking-A-Fast, which is the absence of food for a period of time, in this case over night. When the body does not intake nourishment for a period of time digestion reduces and when food is ingested it take some time for the body to process the food. It is like your car in the wintertime, if you live in an area of the world where there is snow and cold winters, it takes a few minutes for the car to warm up before you get heat and the automobile is able to perform at its optimum levels. The body is no different, it too has to go through a process of warming up in order for the digestive tract to function at its optimum. Many people jump-start their body and digestion with coffee, which wakes up the body and quicken digestion as it opens the lungs (only if the coffee is black without sugar).

Because diabetes is a digestive disorder that reduces the ability of the body to break down food, absorb and assimilate nutrients from that food. It makes it hard for the digestive tract to jump start in the morning when heavy foods are consumed. It takes most peoples digestive tract until mid day to peak and be ready for a heavy meal, so you know a diabetic's digestive tract is going to take longer. Weight gain seen in type 2 diabetics has to do with mal-absorption of nutrients creating accumulation of waste by products in the small intestine. When the body is unable to digest the heavy breakfast of the morning and there is no exercise and the digestive tract is already compromised, then the body will not receive nutrients and there will be a feeling of tiredness, sluggishness and the mind will not be sharp. This is also why many people who eat a heavy breakfast in the morning drink coffee. The caffeine in the coffee acts as digestive stimulant even though some persons feel heavy after eating their breakfast. The stimulant increases their ability to be alert for 2 to 3 hours before they feel sluggish and then reach for sweets or another cup of coffee to wake them up again. This is part of what is causing diabetes and other health disparities.

I suggest diabetics eat light in the morning with maybe whole grain toast, a piece of fruit that is in season, or bowl of oatmeal (oats are a stimulant to the blood sugar and will not raise the levels, as a matter of fact it will assist in the decrease of the blood sugar levels because of the chromium.). These foods will not spike up the blood sugar levels very high and when taken with digestive enzymes these foods assist in proper digestion promoting healthy food to blood sugar levels. The other suggestion is to eat green foods in the morning like green vegetables or a green salad, even a green apple will get you started without complications. This does sound strange; however, many of the diabetics who have tried this have been able to balance their blood sugar levels throughout the day.

This does not cause the body to feel heavy, nor does it cause any bowel issues, as a matter of fact it increase the ability of the bowels to move more frequently when the food is roughage. This roughage is fiber that sweeps the intestinal tract slowly introducing sugar into the blood stream assisting the interaction between the cells, insulin, and glucose uptake. Chlorophyll in green foods is blood builders, blood detoxifiers, promoting circulation, and oxygen to nourish blood and body. In his book "The Healing Power of Chlorophyll from Plant Life" the late Dr. Bernard Jensen stated "In case of diabetes, improving such conditions demands a constant watch of the blood sugar and urine. The addition of chlorophyll will in the long run allow the patient to cut down on insulin, orinase, and other drugs." He goes on to discuss a case where the person's blood sugar was 380 and in three months with the use of chlorophyll it dropped to 118. Chlorophyll maintains healthy blood sugar levels as it provides energy to the body. In the wake of this you will be able to eat two or three meals a day without the drop in blood sugar levels in between meals.

The largest meal of the day should be consumed during lunch because you are able to work it off and assist the glucose to work into the blood over the period from lunch to dinner (dinner should be light meal). At lunch you should have a protein in the form of broiled, baked or rotisserie chicken or fish. You should never eat anything fried. Also a salad made of green foods (dandelion greens, spinach, endives, green string beans a blood sugar lower, Jerusalem artichoke, etc) should be a main attraction during lunch especially in the spring and summer when there are more fresh greens available. Note: the green should have a slight bitter taste to them because they will improve the liver's function and assist in maintaining a healthy blood sugar level. There should be a small bowl of whole grain or a sandwich made from whole grain bread and it would be good to have greens on the sandwich, because the more chlorophyll you receive increases your benefit for the uptake of glucose.

Your dinner meal should not be heavy, chicken or fish and if you eat red meat it should be only about an ounce. The key element here is your need for the meal to digest before going to bed, reducing the time it is sitting in your intestinal tract. Meat can take up to 8 or more hours to digest depending on the method in which it was prepared, chewed, and how it was combined with other foods. Dinner should be eaten by seven o clock at the lattest and consist of some type of green vegetable, whole grain (very little). The whole grain should not be in the form of pasta, bread, or any heavy whole food. You want to make sure the food does not increase your blood sugar levels to where they are high in the morning. You also don't want to feel bloated when you go to sleep.

Always take enzymes with food for better digestion. You will notice your bowel habits improve and the heavy feeling after meals disappear.

I suggest you work within the compounds of the Glycemic Index using food low on the index to balance out your meals. Purchase cookbooks and modify the recipe to fit your blood sugar levels. Be very careful about how you add foods to you regiment and always check the index before eating a food. If you work with the index and the suggestion made in this book you will find your glucose levels decrease along with the medication as your body becomes nourished as you over come Mal-absorption, and malnutrition.

QI Gong

"Discipline of the body works to discipline your mind. Discipline your mind and you strengthen your body."

Grandmaster Tae Yun Kim
The Silent Master Awakening the Power Within

Studies have shown there is a need for exercise within the entire country, especially amongst overweight and obese people who are at great risk for type 2 diabetes. Physical activity assists in the promotion of blood circulation, reduction in adiposity, and decreases cholesterol and has been known to aid diabetics in eliminating diabetic's medication.[180] Exercise promotes the uptake of glucose into the cells by GLUT-4 transporters, which is the same method used by insulin.

When a diabetic develops a consistent exercise program they begin to see weight loss and their fasting blood sugar levels decrease, along with an increase in energy. A good exercise program is preformed at least three times a week for 30 minutes to an hour per session. The exercise does not have to be heavy or vigorous, but steady and consistent. Some diabetics choose to run which is okay however; they have to run on a surface that is gentle on their knees. In this case treadmill, grass, a track, or Astor turfs are good surfaces to run on. Many people in the United States are adopting exercises from China, and India like Yoga, Tai Chi, and Qi Gong. All of these exercises are aerobic exercises in nature even though they are slow standing and seating postures. I have found them to be effective with diabetics. They open the joints, promote blood flow, increase movement in the lower abdomen improving bowel function, and invigorating the entire body.

Qi Gong (pronounced chee-gung) is part of Traditional Chinese exercise system consisting of breathing, easy in some cases light exercise postures to increase the flow of Qi, blood and body fluids and also including meditation. It open, stretches and develops muscles, tendons and ligaments as it improves your inner awareness and promotes longevity. Just as there are many different styles of Tai Chi, there are also different styles of Qi Gong and it is known by may names (chi kung, chi gong, chi gung, and daoyin). China Healthways International concludes more than 1.3 million people in Beijing China practice some form of Qigong every day, where throughout China Qigong is practiced by more than 80 million people.[181]

The Asian population practice Qigong for health and longevity and not as a sport. In his book Chinese Medical Qigong Therapy A Comprehensive Clinical Text, Dr. Jerry Alan Johnson, writes "Qigong is the skillful practice of gathering, circulating, and applying life-force energy." He goes on to state," Medical Qigong therapy is the oldest of the four branches of Traditional Chinese Medicine and provides the energetic foundation from which acupuncture, herbal healing, and Chinese massage originates. It is through the understanding of Qigong that the other branches of Traditional Chinese Medicine are elevated to a spiritual path of self-realization and internal transformation."[182]

In his statements Dr. Johnson points out several factors needed in the healing of diabetes, overweight and obese people. In his description he uses the terms gathering, and circulating. Gathering means pulling together the inner resources needed for the body to balance its self (blood, body fluid, Qi). Once achieved, then these elements circulate through the body with the movement of Qi, promoting life to cells, tissues, organs and systems and in the process reducing and/or eliminating diabetes and other health disparities. This 5000 year old exercise system has shown to eliminate toxins from the body, restore energy, reduce stress, anxiety and improve the uptake of glucose according to Queensland Qigong Program, funded by the Diabetes Australia Research Trust, conducted at University Queensland Australia, School of Human Movement Studies lead by Professor Wendy Brown and researcher Dr. Yvette Miller and Dr. Nicola Burton.[183]

Throughout the United States there are many schools, certified practitioners who are qualified to lead you through Medical Qigong for diabetes. There is a difference between medical qigong and qigong. A Medical Qigong instructor has knowledge of the medical Chinese system where he/she can guide you through Qigong exercise to directly address your illness (diabetes). An instructor who is only instructed in Qigong could be very well versed in Qigong, but not the medical side of Chinese medicine in order to directly assist in the healing of diabetes. However, either form of Qigong will provide you with some improvement in your blood sugar levels.

A Traditional Chinese Medical look at healing Diabetes

"Life is depending on you to shine. Life is waiting on you to bloom. Life is waiting on you to glorify it. Please don't let life down."

Iyanla Vanzant
Faith in the Valley

My background is in nutrition, herbs and Chinese Medicine. I could not complete this book without touching on Traditional Chinese Medicine (TCM) and its influence in reversing diabetes. TCM views diabetes very much different than allopathic medicine (medicine practiced in US hospitals). It works with the root cause of the disease and not the symptoms. Through the evaluation of the tongue, pulse, and body palpation, the doctor is able to assess the root of the disorder and recommend a remedy that will work to address the cause. Diabetes is a heat related disorder in TCM and is caused by stomach heat. However, there are many other different root causes as you will see later. Everyone who has diabetes is not treated the same, because each person is an individual and has to be treated as one. This is why TCM is able to reverse diabetes and assist the person in maintaining their health and longevity.

I have attempted to break down the information to a level where you can understand it, because I know it is foreign to you and the concepts are not your everyday ones. You will also find the nourishing and controlling charts that will guide you through the stages of understanding the methodology I am working with here to express my point. You will also find footnotes on terms I think you are not familiar with. TCM is easy to understand and work with once you have grasped the concept behind the work.

Understanding the Emotional Boundaries of Diabetes through Traditional Chinese Medicine (TCM)

Diabetes is referred to as Xiao Ke (wasting and thirsting), xiao dan (pure heat wasting), ge xiao (diaphragm wasting), xiao zhong (central wasting).[184] The references made in the NeiJing Suwen the oldest traditional Chinese medical (TCM) book still in existence. The explanation of this concept lends itself not only to the physiology of the organs, but to the energy, and emotional balance of the organs. TCM views the disease with a concept far beyond western medicine level of thinking. Looking at it from a Chinese perspective it comes in depth, as TCM looks for the root cause of the dis-ease and not just at the symptoms. I am going to put limitations on this section of the book only because I could write an entire volume on diabetes and Chinese medicine. The concepts of TCM have to really be understood and that take time. It took me over twenty years to really grasp many of the concepts of TCM. I would like for you to have an idea for another type of medicine that has addressed diabetes with success in reducing and eliminating it and the complications that come with diabetes. Oriental Asian have a particular way of living and only when they become westernized are they unable to heal from diseases. Their eating habits, their culture is all part of health and healing. When I was in China studying almost every one you saw had a thermos filled with some type of tea. As a matter of fact, Dr. Wang would not allow us to start class without drinking tea. We look at it as tea, but for over 6,000 or more years Asian people practice health through their daily herbal tea.

In order for you to understand the Chinese system I must first take you through a few concepts and systems. One of the systems is the organ network. The Chinese organ system views the organs as a network that is inter-connected to each other. What effects one set of organs creates an affect to another set of organs. The organs are married to each other, with a mother/child and grandparent/grandchild relationship, also known as the nourishing and controlling cycles in TCM. If one set of organs is strong then it can nourish its child and control the activity of its grandchild, as it builds the body and balance the emotions. On the other hand, if the set of organs are weak then it can cause its child to be weak and it will attach the organs (grandchild) it controls creating instability in the network resulting in health issues.

The organ network is very powerful when it comes to healing the body, mind, spirit. Their connection balances each other and relies on each other for the needed Qi, nutrients and fluids to maintain health and well being. There are times when the mother organ will have to be treated to balance the child and vise versa. In other cases the grandchild has to be treated to maintain the balance of the grandparent.

The network relationship is as follows the liver (LV) is married to the gallbladder (GB) and nourishes the heart/small intestine (HT/SI). LV/GB controls the spleen/stomach/pancreas (SP/ST/PA). HT/SI nourishes the (SP/ST/PA) and controls the lungs/large intestine (LU/LI). SP/ST/PA nourishes the LU/LI and controls the kidney/bladder (KD/BL). The LU/LI nourishes the KD/BL and controls the LV/GB. The KD/BL nourishes the LV/GB and controls the HT/SI. Refer to the two charts below for the flow and direction in which this connection moves.

Attached to this are physical, emotional, and spiritual attributes. I will deal with the emotional balance of the organ network and its relationship to diabetes. In western medicine the focus is always on the physiological aspect of the disease and not the emotion that could be the back bone of the organs failing. In traditional Chinese medicine they say "disease comes from the seven emotions, *worry, grief, fear, anger, pensiveness, anxiety, and sadness*." In my practice I discuss with my clients' their emotional relationship with diabetes, which provides an understanding of not having to change their eating habits, exercise and think healthy thoughts, but they have to check their emotional status as well. Each organ houses an emotion that is positive or negative depending on which one a person uses more will depend on how their health will develop. Western medicine is beginning to investigate the relationship between a persons' mental attitude and their health, where the Chinese have used this intervention for over 6,000 years. For instance western medicine is now looking at the affect of meditation on heart disease. As we know, meditation calms the mind and creates a balance in the mind for peace and tranquility, which promotes health and well being. Meditation reduces oxidative stress, increasing oxygen to the cells, as it assists the body in removing waste from the body and cells, preventing high blood pressure, heart disease, stroke, cancer, etc.

I will also focus on the climatical conditions that are also associated with the organs because the emotions and the climatical conditions work hand and hand. There is a delicate balance between the two. One will support the other and vise versa. The emotional and climatical condition can also be stimulated by food as well. When discussing climatical conditions, we view it in the same manner as in the atmosphere of the world, cold, wind, dry, hot, damp, heat, wet. All of these conditions occur in the body as they do in nature. Each of them represents an illness that could promote another illness. In TCM, diabetes is a heat related dis-ease mainly of the stomach and can be caused by excessive worrying, or anxiety. Both of these emotions are from the spleen/pancreas/stomach and they can not only cause heat, but dampness as well. When we see dampness it comes in the form of abdominal distention relating to being overweight, which is another cause of diabetes. I have seen cases where a client would work on their physiology (health of the body) and their emotions at the same time and the illness reduced or was eliminated. I have also seen a person work just on the emotions and their health returned.

The chart identifies the organs, their emotions and corresponding areas of the body.

Organs	Emotion	Areas of the body
Lungs/Large intestine	Sadness/Grief	Skin
Kidney/Bladder	Fear/Kindness	Bones/Reproductive organs/Head hair/Brain Marrow
Liver/Gallbladder	Depression/anxiety/anger	Muscles/Eyes
Heart/Small Intestine	Impatience/Joy	Blood vessels/Brain/Spirit
Pericardium/Triple Heater	Impatience/Joy	Blood vessels/Brain/Spirit
Spleen/stomach/pancreas	Anxiety/"Worry"/	Digestion/"Ligaments"/

QI

"By changing ourselves and training our state of life, we advance to changing and adjusting the patterns of life. We should consciously and actively change the patterns of our life and daily life, including the patterns of eating and sleeping, and the pattern of life span."

Dr. Yan Xin
Secrets and Benefits of Internal Qigong Cultivation

Moving on to the next topic is the identification of some terms used in TCM you need to be familiar with. The word Qi (chee) refers to an energy that is the life force of everything and is everywhere and in everything whether it is living or not. According to Wiseman and Ye's second edition of A Practical Dictionary of Chinese Medicine, the word Qi has many different definitions, the one that stands out the most is "Anything of any particular nature." Another definition is "Human growth and development, as well as all physiological activity and metabolism, are manifestations of the activity of qi." It is also said that there is not really any English translation for the word Qi.

There are several other words used in Chinese medicine such as deficiencies, excess, stagnation, balance, and harmony. Deficiency is the lack of or not enough to create balance, which could be Qi, blood or body fluids. Excess means too much, an over abundance. Stagnation is when Qi, blood or body fluids are no longer moving and they are stuck in one place increasing swelling, distention or discoloration. Balance is where Qi, blood or body fluids are equal throughout the body. Harmony is when the body is balanced and there is not dis-ease. It is important for me to note this as we move into the Chinese section of the organ network's relationship to the emotions of Diabetes.

Yin/Yang Concept

Yin is another word that is used throughout Chinese culture, philosophy and medicine. Yin is the balancing principal of yang. It is referred to as the weaker element, darkness, passiveness, water, lower part of the body, the energy falling down, inner movement, night and it is the principal of female. Yang is the stronger element, has a fire principal, rises, is light, aggressive, external movement, upper part of the body, day and its principal is male. I will identify each organ separately and then connect their relationship to the network.

Organ Network

Let me provide you with a brief description of the Chinese organ network so you will have a better understanding of where I am going with this information. The organ network assists in understanding the connection of the organs and how they work to maintain health and well being or create health challenges. I have found this is the only way I can successfully explain and assist a person as their bodies take control to reduce and/or eliminate diabetes. You may ask yourself why this information is important to me? It is important because with it you will have more tools to work with in your quest to assist a family member, a friend or yourself with the ability to reveres the diabetes.

In TCM all of the organs are networking together through a marriage, control and nourishing cycle, as I will explain. Each of these processes governs the balance of the body, mind, and spirit. When the network is out of balance the body displays disharmony and by understanding the workings of the network one is able to assist the body in creating harmony. If we look at physiology of diabetes it is a disharmony of heat causing a wasting of the cells and tissues relating to the stomach. The stomach infringes on the spleen, which impedes on the lungs/large intestines creating breathing problems, and constipation. Now the lungs/large intestine inhibits the kidney/bladder, which increase the ability of the person to have hypertension, fertility issues and polyuria. On the other hand the kidneys infringe on the liver by not providing it with water promoting heat and stagnation of Qi, and blood resulting in high blood pressure, elevated cholesterol, and temperamental issues of depression, anxiety. The liver then impedes on the heart/small intestine, which increase the person's risk of heart dis-ease, stroke, elevated cholesterol and weight gain. As I have pointed out when one organ is in disharmony, it can take the entire network with it. This is the method in which Chinese therapists view the body and health issues.

As I stated the organs are married to one another, for instance, the liver is married to the gallbladder, the heart to the small intestine, the spleen/pancreas to the stomach, the lungs to the large intestine, and the kidney to the bladder. (See the chart) This only means that anything that affects one organ in the marriage affects the other. Each of the organs promotes a different emotion that either weakens them or strengthens them. When the emotion weakens the organ it then is able to create disharmonies that result in disease. Let's take a look at the organs and their emotions, which will provide you with some insight on your relationship to the emotion and diabetes.

The chart provides you with a visual graphic idea of the information I just explained. In my example I only explained the Nourishing cycle. The controlling cycle is similar and works in the same manner.

Nourishing Cycle

When an organ nourishes (mother) another organ (child) the nourishing organ provides the needed balance for the organ it is nourishing. Only if the mother organ is strong can it provide the child organ with what it needs to maintain its balance. On the other hand, if the mother organ is weak than it will be unable to provide the child with healing energy and may begin to take energy from the child rendering the child weak and unable to carry out its function.

Controlling Cycle

The controlling cycle is much different in the controlling organs; as like grandparents and the organ they are controlling are like grandchildren. The controlling organ (grandparent) make sure the controlled organ (grandchild) has the needed energy to carry out their function, when the grandparent is weak they will attack the grandchild, making the child weak and creating disharmonies.

An example in diabetes:

If a person has a lot of frustration, which is a liver condition, and does not resolve the issues over a period of time, their liver becomes over heated and starts to attack the spleen and stomach the result is an impaired digestion, absorption, assimilation, and improper elimination leading to the sweet cravings. These sweet cravings become hypoglycemic in nature (low blood sugar) where over time they become hyperglycemia (diabetes). This happens because the frequent ingesting of sugar weakens the spleen/pancreas to the point where spleen Qi (energy) and stomach yin (water) are depleted resulting in the burnout and diabetes results. The other part of that is the sugar begins to store in the body as dampness (mucus/phlegm) and moves into the abdomen where it accumulates and weight gain occurs. Then, it creates a risk of over weight conditions, obesity and/or type 2 diabetes. This has occurred because of one organ in the network being emotionally out of balance. In TCM, every thing we do accounts for how well our health will be and what is needed to reduce and/or eliminate the issues at hand.

Most of the time with diabetic, in TCM there is an issue with the digestive tract including the spleen/pancreas/stomach. In traditional Chinese medicine the pancreas is not really recognized. The spleen takes it place as one of the major digestive organs, which is not like the role the spleen plays in western medicine where the spleen is just a lymphatic organ and receive used red blood cells. It is very much the opposite, working with the stomach, which decides what is food and what is a waste by product. The spleen takes the ripe (usable nutrients) and distributes nutrients through the body and then creates blood.

Traditional Organ Network Chart

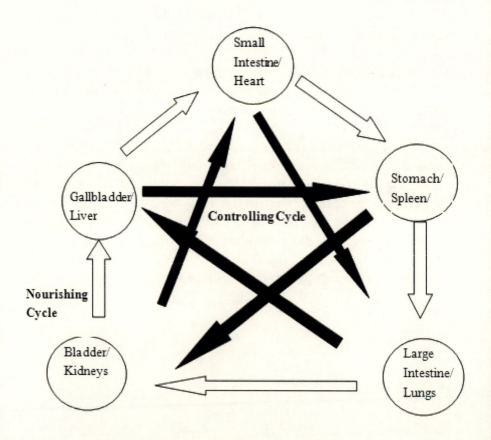

Traditional Chinese Organ Network

"Life forms are stations for the reception and transmission of forces, through which all are nourished. Each thing exists to nourish all others and, in return, to be nourished and transmit life."

Vasant Lad and David Frawely
The Yoga of Herbs

Liver/Gallbladder

The liver and gallbladder are nourished by the kidney/bladder and are controlled by the lungs/large intestine. The liver/gallbladder in return nourish the heart/small intestine and control the activity of the spleen and stomach. The liver/gallbladder are the organs most likely to become excessive. In other words become stagnated, creating heat and attacking other organs. This mean the live/gallbladder are the most likely organs to cause other health issues because of their instability. The inabilities they can cause are gas pains, menstrual disorders, digestive imbalance, chest tightness and/or pain, etc. The emotions of these organs include anger, frustration, anxiety, suppression, and depression. They rule over the muscles, and the liver stores the blood.

Liver

The liver has a very different job in TCM than in Western medicine. It not only provides physiological conditions it also provides energetically ones as well. The Liver is the General of the body it makes sure all the functions of the body are running smooth as it stores blood and make sure the entire body functions well. It is able to restore depleted Qi (energy) to the rest of the body if it is healthy and well and not in a hyper (excessive) mode. In his book "Dragon Rises, Red Bird Flies," Dr. Leon Hammer, states "Functionally, the Liver is especially endowed in that, according to Chinese medicine, it "stores the blood". Rich in blood, the Liver is more capable of restoring itself than any other organ system. In fact, one of its most important functions for the entire body lies in recovering all the energy when the body is depleted." [185] The sensory organ of the Liver is the eyes (diabetic blindness) and it controls the nervous system (neuropathy). Its emotions include anger, suppression, depression, frustration, repression, resentment, anxiety and it houses tension and stress. All of these emotions affect the blood, its stability levels and its ability to flow through the body. The body parts that the Liver rules are ligaments, muscles and tendons.

Traumas, tingling and numbness (neuropathy) can stem from an issue with Liver blood being low, stagnated and/or not circulating in the body. In many cases a person with diabetes may be in a stressful or other emotional situation (job, family, friend, etc) causing the Liver to develop into a hyper state where the blood is not circulating (stagnated) and creating tingling and numbness in the extremities.

Dr. Hammer states "The sub-syndrome, deficiency of yin of the Liver may cause hyperactivity of the Liver yang, which turns into fire and ascends to the top or invades the channels and Collaterals,[xxi] causing mental confusion and hemiplegia.[xxii] The Liver also manifests what is

---

[xxi] Collaterals (Luo) The body's energy streams that branch off the Twelve Primary Channels and the Conceptional and Governing Vessels. Johnson J, A. Ph.D, D.T.C.M., D.M.Q. Chinese Medical Qigong Therapy A Comprehensive Clinical Text.

[xxii] Hemiplegia: total or partial paralysis of one side of the body that results from disease of or injury to the moter centers of the brain. Merriam Webster's Medical Desk Dictionary, Revised Edition, Springfield, Massachusttes, USA.

known as wind. With deficiency of the blood of the Liver, the tendons can no longer be nourished; with the stirring of the Liver wind causes numbness of the extremities, tremor, and convulsions.

It is stated in the Chinese medical system that there are five earthly elements that govern the body. Each of the organ systems corresponds to one of these elements that also have climate conditions. In this case the Liver is related to wind. Wind is an element that moves in the body like it blows around on the earth moving things from one place to another. It happens the same way in the body. As a matter of fact, wind and Qi are responsible for the movement of energy moving through the nervous system. Many people with diabetes have emotional issues that are not factored into the equation of the disease and these emotional issues don't have to be severe but just enough to cause the liver to become hyperactive. Any time a person is under stress that is an emotional imbalance the Liver has to deal with. When the emotions (depression, anger, stress, etc) are out of balance it inhibits the free flow of Qi creating toxic energy, which develops into heat and expands into wind. This wind now reduces the Liver's ability to detoxify causing tension in the muscles (cramps and/or spasms) including the heart (the heart is also a muscle) resulting in the blood pressure elevating (hypertension—lack of magnesium and potassium to relax the heart). Wind is also responsible for strokes (TCM calls it "Wind Stroke"), paralysis of one side of the body, deviation of the mouth or eye like in Bells Palsy. Heat in the Liver causes it to become stagnated (excessiveness—hyperactivity) reducing the Liver's ability to properly store blood. Now the Liver is unable to buffer the glucose complex resulting in hypoglycemia (low blood sugar) and many type of allergic reactions.[186] This also results in weight gain because the Liver controls the activity of the Spleen/Stomach/Pancreas. These are the primary factors of the digestive system in TCM. The Liver attacking the Spleen/Stomach/Pancreas reduces their ability to function properly resulting in heat and dampness in these organs and the making of type 2 diabetes.

When the Liver is in heat or a state of stagnation it reduces the production of bile, which decreases the flow of bile to the gallbladder. Over working the Liver causing less bile to be secreted into the small intestine reducing the movement of the bowels and increases the stagnation of waste by products in the small intestine. The end result in abdominal is distention and weight gain.

Gallbladder

The Gallbladder is an interesting organ because it is considered a bowel, however, it does not store, transport or come in contact with food, drink or waste by products and never comes directly in contact with any of the external digestive components (mouth, rectum or anus). On the other hand, it does in its capacity as a bowel, stores bile, which it receives from the liver and then secrets it into the small intestine promoting bowel movements. The composition of bile salts includes electrolytes, bile pigments (Bilirubin), cholesterol, and other fatty acids. It assists in the elimination of excessive cholesterol and the degrading of worn out red blood cells. One of bile's major jobs is to emulsify fatty acids making them usable by the body and increase the ability of the fat-soluble vitamins to be absorbed into the body. This is why in Chinese medicine it is referred to as one of the six ordinary organs. It is a yang organ, but acts like a yin organ because of its storing capacity.

A large percentage of people with diabetes also have high cholesterol. Some of them also have gallstones and have their gallbladders removed, which according to traditional Chinese medicine creates imbalance affecting their mental and emotion states of being. When a person's gallbladder is remove, they find their self being very indecisive, problems planning their life, and their judgment is off.

Heart/Small Intestine

In the organ network the next set of organs is the Heart/Small Intestine. They are nourished by the Liver/Gallbladder and are affected by the balance of these two organs. If the Liver shows signs of stress, anger, depression, irritation, or frustration it's affects on the heart can cause the mind to lack joy, happiness and weaken the blood reducing the bloods ability to flow promoting cardiovascular disease and in some case arthrosclerosis. On the other hand, when the heart is negatively influenced by the liver the blood and Qi is unable to circulate to the extremities they become cold, numb and result in neuropathy and/or a leg sore that develops into gangrene promoting amputation of limbs as seen with many diabetic. Because diabetes is a blood disease this factor is of importance.

Heart

The emotions of the person play a large part of their healing process. The heart is very sensitive in the emotion of joy and patience. Humans are creatures of pleasure and entertainment. This creates a factor for the joy and when that joy is not there we find our self in another space and our health begins to show the lack of this emotion. The other side of this is that when there is too much joy it can also cause the same type of imbalances. If a person seems to have an abundance of joy they could find their self having insomnia and being impatient. In many case the emotion of joy is lacking, affecting the temperament causing stagnation of blood, weaken the hearts ability to promote an even blood flow to the entire body. The emotion of the Heart/Small Intestine is joy. The heart governs blood through circulation, as it controls the activities of the blood vessels, houses the mind, and maintains the health of the complexion and controls sweating. The heart is also the home of the spirit. When the heart is deficient the blood is unable to circulate creating coldness of the hands and feet, dullness of the mind, fatigue, insomnia and impatience. One of the things seen in people who are over weight is they tend to spontaneously sweat or they are excessively warm, which is a heart Qi deficiency. This has bearings on how the heart controls the activity of the lungs/large intestine, which controls the opening and closing of the pores. Also Heart/Small Intestine nourishes the spleen/stomach/pancreas, which are the organs of digestion.

Small Intestine

The Small Intestines is one of the most powerful organs in the body and the most misunderstood. In most cases the doctor refers to it as your stomach so most of us think it is our stomach, especially when it is distended. The small intestines is the warehouse for the exchange from food (Gu Qi—food essence) to nutrients. It absorbs the nutrients and integrates them into the body where they nourish the cells, tissues and organs. On an other note the Small Intestine separates the waste by products from the food and directs it to the Large Intestine and Bladder to be expelled out of the body. In Chinese medicine the Small Intestine is referred to as " The Official in Charge of Separating the Pure from the Impure."

In type 2 diabetes we see that the Small Intestine plays a major role, and yet it is not really addressed. The Small Intestine is the beginning site of overweight and obese conditions. It is where the waste by products of the food is stored on its way to the Large Intestine and Bladder. In the case of weight gain, or should I say waste gain, the Small Intestine is unable to complete its cycle and the waste becomes trapped and accumulates in the Small Intestine where it leaks into the blood stream resulting in health conditions including diabetes, hypertension, elevated cholesterol, etc.

Physicians suggest their overweight diabetic patients go on a diet. The fact is diets do not work, because they address the symptoms and not the real problem. They work well as long as the person is on the diet, when the person returns to eating the foods they once ate or stop eating the manufactured food of the program the weight returns with a vengeance. As I pointed out in an earlier section one of the issues with diabetics is constipation and the Small Intestine is the main site. It is where we have to begin in order to reduce and/or eliminate overweight and obese conditions in relationship to diabetes and other health issues.

I have found by presenting a person with a healthy lifestyle program they tend to lose the waste, reduce their weight and their blood sugar levels decrease. The sweet craving diminish, they have more energy, and they think clearer. They also feel free and easy and better about their ability to do the work they do in society.

Emotionally, the Small Intestine represents the ability to think clearly and distinguish the balance of issues when making a decision. It aids in balancing out thought patterns, where the gallbladder has to do with the decision itself and the spleen has to do with the thought the Small Intestine deals with the pattern of both decision and thoughts and how the emotions of them affect the person.

Spleen/Stomach/Pancreas

The Spleen/Stomach/Pancreas (in TCM the pancreas is not recognized, the spleen takes the place of the pancreas.) are the major digestive organs and the primary site of diabetes, although the lungs, liver and kidneys are also involved. The stomach receives the food and discriminates which part of the food is ripe and which is rotten. The ripe portion is transported to the spleen where it is transformed into nutrients, blood and is transported through the body for nourishment. The spleen in TCM does not perform the same function as in Western medicine. It manufactures blood, red blood cells, and transforms and transports nutrients throughout the body. It also promotes the development of Qi, the vital energy of all forms whether alive or not alive. A person who has diabetes has low energy because the spleen lacks the ability to promote blood in a manner where it invigorates the body. When the Spleen is weak and vacuous it is not able to extract the Qi (energy/nutrients) from food, leaving a person tired and in need of something to boost their energy (sweets). The taste of the Spleen/Stomach is sweet, that is why sweets and refined carbohydrates have such a devastating impact on people with hyperglycemia (high blood sugar) and hypoglycemia (low blood sugar). It is ironic how diabetics know they should not have sweets and they can't stay away from sweets.

There are also a large number of people in the world who are predisposed to diabetes because they have hypoglycemia where they consume sweets several times during the day to maintain a energy level that aids them in making it through the day. They are unaware of the Spleen/Stomach being overworked, which can not only result in diabetes, but other diseases like Candida, elevated cholesterol, neurological conditions, etc. It also impacts on the emotions of the person reducing their ability to concentrate, nervous energy and thinking too much. As a matter of fact many diabetics find their self with insomnia because they can not shut down their minds at night or they have polyuria and are unable to return to sleep because their thoughts are constantly penetrating their minds. In some case the person is always worrying about something. Excessive worrying, anxiety, and over thinking damage the Spleen/Stomach and are the basis for diabetes.

Spleen

When the Spleen is weak/vacuous it is susceptible to dampness (phlegm and mucus build up) and dampness as in the atmosphere is heavy and dull. Dampness is heavy and sinks to the abdomen where it accumulates in the small intestine resulting in abdominal distention and increases weight gain, as well as waste leaking into the blood causing cholesterol and other health problems. This can come from several factors, 1) the consumption of too many saturated fats, which are damp by nature, 2) over eating too many refined sugars in the form of processed carbohydrates and sweet foods, 3) foods that are overcooked and processed, 4) drinking and eating at the same meal, and 5) eating under emotional stress. At any rate it calculates to the development of health conditions such as overweight, obesity and diabetes.

Sweet foods damage the spleen as noted in the book The Treatment of Diabetes Mellitus with Chinese Medicine where it states, "Dampness in the Spleen damages it, leading to both its encumbrance and vacuity." It goes on to say "in Chinese medicine, it is believed that the sweet flavor is moderated or relaxing. Therefore, persons experiencing liver depression and/or Qi stagnation typically crave sweets as a sort of self-medication of their tension and depression. While sweet-flavored foods may temporarily relax this tension and depression, ultimately they damage the spleen." [187] The Su Wen (Simple Questions) Treatise on Strange Disease," Say, This [condition] occurs in those who are fat and beautiful. This person must [eat] many sweet, fine [foods] and too many fats. Fats all cause heat inside humans, and sweets all cause center fullness. Therefore, the Qi spills over above, transforming into wasting and thirsting."[188] The inter-operation of this passage is when a person consumes too many fats and sweet foods the sweet foods create dampness (mucus, phlegm) and that settles in the region of the abdomen creating distention (type 2 overweight condition). The fats create heat that rises into the stomach, (creating a counter flow of its energy) and producing heat, which promotes thirst that most diabetic have. We do find people who are suffering from depression to consume an abundance of either sweets or fatty foods to comforted their self.

Spleen dampness can turn to damp heat descending to the pelvis causing impotence, (many diabetic males experience), restless leg syndrome, leg sores, urinary disturbances, and vaginitis.[189] I have seen diabetic women in my practice with yeast overgrowth (Candida), and/or vaginal yeast infections, especially if they are overweight. As well, there have been men who have had impotent problems because of the diabetes and/or overweight condition with Candida in conjunction with diabetes. The Spleen does not like dampness and encourages dryness, where the stomach does not like dryness and encourages dampness.

Stomach

The Stomach is very important in the manufacturing of diabetes from a traditional Chinese medicine prospective, because when there is stomach heat and dryness the risk of diabetics increases. As a matter of fact, stomach heat can acerbate fluids causing dryness resulting in the thirst most diabetics encounter. The heat increases the body's wasting condition resulting in a reduction of organ moisture increasing dryness affecting the stomach's rotten and ripping process, inhibiting body nourishment. In this capacity the stomach becomes imbalanced and invades the kidneys resulting in polyuria increasing the dryness and wasting. This attack on the kidneys increase the risk of renal failure, which is the end result for many diabetics, where it increases the stress on the kidneys to the point where the person has to undertake dialysis or they die from kidney failure.

The kidneys are the major water organs of the body, where the lungs make sure the organs have moisture. The Spleen/Stomach nourish the Lungs/Large Intestine, when there is diabetes the Spleen/Stomach are unable to nourish their child Lung/Large Intestine, inhibiting their function decreasing the ability of the lungs to moisten the organ network and reduces the large intestines ability to eliminate waste (constipation is a result of bowel dryness, which the bowels need moisture to be fluent). It also hinders the Lungs/Large Intestine protective Qi (immunity) function (I will talk more on this next). The heat of diabetes causes body fluids to dry up and without the nourishment of the fluids the body waste away. We have to remember the body is three quarters water.

Lungs

When we think about the lungs, we think about breathing and how they allow us to take in air and release carbon monoxide into the atmosphere. TCM views the lungs in the same manner, however, there is a difference in their philosophy as the Lungs/Large Intestines promote Wei Qi or the protective element of the body known in Western medicine as the immune system. The Qi patrols the surface of the skin protecting the body from external pathogenic influences. The protective Qi of the Large Intestines/ Lungs is able to assist the body in its ability to harmonize food Qi (energy) from the Spleen. In other words lung Qi assists the body in receiving nutrients from food as it penetrates and nourishes the body to ward off disease and maintain health. It would reduce and/or eliminate any wasting process within the body and as diabetes is known as a wasting disease.

In type 1 diabetes where a child has consumed cow's milk or formula, which breaks down their immune system, they often suffer from colds, runny nose, constipation and ear infections. This is because the lungs Qi is deficient and the body is unable to be protected by lung Qi. This sets the stage for the distraction of the alpha and beta cells resulting in type 1 diabetes. When Lung Qi is deficient it is unable to descend and the Qi blocks the chest and produces cough, dry mouth, hoarseness, and scanty sticky phlegm.

One of the jobs of the lungs is to maintain the waterways. This means to make sure all the organs are moist and are able to maintain moisture. When Lung Qi becomes deficient they are unable to assist other organs in maintaining their moisture resulting in dryness, dry mouth, thirst, and polyuria. In some cases the person will have frequent coughs and colds or have year round allergies. This Lung Qi deficiency can be caused by Stomach, which is in an excessive mode, creating heat that invades the Lungs/Large Intestines reducing the Lungs ability to promote fluids and affecting its counterpart the Large Intestine resulting in constipation, which later can transform into abdominal distention, elevated cholesterol, increased blood pressure and type 2 diabetes. The liver can also cause Lung Qi not to descend or move in its natural downward flow, resulting in tightness in the chest and cough.

Lung Qi along with Heart Qi promotes the movement of blood, body fluid, and circulates these elements throughout the body. This would also make the lungs responsible for the blood transportation to the extremities and when Lung Qi is unable to promote this movement, then there is numbness and tingling of the extremities. Even though the liver houses the blood, the lungs move the blood through the channels and vessels. On the other hand the heart control the blood vessels and Lung Qi promotes the flow of the blood through the vessels. In its role as the child of the spleen, the Lungs aid the spleen in its ability to transform and transport food (Zhong Qi) nutrients and circulate it throughout the body.

The emotional imbalance of Lungs Qi is from sadness, grief, and worry. Worrying affects the chest cavity disallowing Lung Qi to descend creating tension and stagnation in the chest. Again this will impact the large intestine where it is unable to function properly, causing abdominal distention promoting constipation, along with gasping for breath and in some cases sweating. The Lung is responsible for the opening and closing of the pores. In most cases sweating is related to the Lungs, however, when there is spontaneous sweating the heart is involved. This body reaction is seen in many diabetics who are overweight.

The Lungs are inhibited by the emotions of sadness, worry and grief. As we know worry is an empty emotion, because nine times out of ten the thing we are worried about does not come out the way we worry about it. There are those times when the concept of the worry comes out the way we worry about the situation. Worry binds and knots Qi creating a lump in your throat, heaviness of the chest, difficulty breathing. It is stated "Qi stagnation in the chest deriving from worry may also affect the breast in women and it is often at the root of the formation of breast lumps."[190]

Lung Qi is depleted by sadness and grief resulting in shortness of breath and tightness in the chest. In his book "Dragon Rise Red Bird Flies," Leon Hammer, MD states" Sadness concerns an unresolved, and most often unconscious, early experience of Grief." He goes on to say, "Because grief is usually expressed by crying and sobbing, the breathing apparatus at the physiological level is heavily involved in the reaction of sadness. To control the outward expression of sadness, one has to suppress the breathing mechanism. For this reason, sadness at first affects the lungs, likewise lung disease can lead to unexplained sadness." [191]

The physiological aspect of grief on the Lungs in Traditional Chinese Medicine is its power over the digestive tract, where it digests excessive mucus produced by the Stomach and Spleen. This often occurs from poor eating habits where the Spleen is weak and is unable to transfer and transform food into nutrients. Grief creates upper respiratory issues that affect the heart resulting in epilepsy, dysphagia (difficulty in swallowing), and stroke. Excessive phlegm causes obstructions in the brain (phlegm misting the mind) resulting in a stroke, which then is connected to the Liver and Kidney's energies promoting hypertension as the Spleen and Stomach promotes overweight and obese, eventually developing into diabetes.[192]

Large Intestine

The Large intestine receives the waste products of the food and drink from the small intestine before expelling this waste out of the body. In it's function the large intestine reabsorbs water for the fecal matter back into the body. This is carried out by wave like motion of muscle contraction within the intestine known as peristalsis (Qi movement). Whenever Qi is stagnated it interrupts the flow of the large intestine resulting in constipation, that affects the small intestine and displays itself as abdominal distention. You will find 95.9% of type 2 diabetics abdomen distended. I often explain to people the fact that even if your bowels move two or three times a day, if your abdomen is distended then you are constipated because the fecal matter you see may be from two or three or more months, year ago. This is why the bowel has such a foul smell. The body should not have an offensive smell, in fact you should not smell the bowel at all. The smell is only because the waste has accumulated in the small and large intestines for such a long period of time.

When the large intestine is in disharmony, it causes the lung disharmony. The lungs are very instrumental in the movement of the bowels. Whenever the lung Qi is deficient it inhibits the large intestines ability to pass bowels and if the large intestine is stagnated then it inhibits the downward motion of lung Qi given rise to breathlessness.[193] This is seen in diabetic and people who are overweight. Many times you see them gasping for breath and in some cases they have to stop walking for a minute to gather their breath. Obese people find their self spontaneously sweating, a direct result of the pores not closing and water (yin) being released from the body. As I have stated the skin is the sensory organ of the lungs and large intestine. The impact of the large intestine stagnation not only affects diabetes and its risks, but also increasing the prevalence of high blood pressure, elevated cholesterol, bowel and other dis-eases.

Many people who have diabetes find some point in their life a sadness that they won't let go of and they carry it around with them. Not letting go of people, places issues, and things builds up in the body creating stagnation (constipation of the mind) to where it develops into a comfort zone that you refuse to step out of because the fear (kidney emotion) of what may be on the outside of that comfort zone is greater than your faith (kidney) in you and your spirit. For instance, as a diabetic you live with the reality of being a diabetic all your life because medical science has told you there is not cure for diabetes. Your fear of trying anything new that could possibly improve your health is not in your life plan. The interesting thing is some people do step outside of that zone, and when they see it working they become afraid of it working and revert back to their old behaviors. Now there are those diabetics who have stepped out of their zone and have reversed their diabetes and have not returned to old habits. In many cases diabetics are so set in their comfort zone that they won't even change their eating habits to see if their diabetes improves. The large intestine is about letting go.

Kidney

The kidneys are referred to as the Root of Life in Traditional Chinese Medicine (TCM). This means they are the foundation of life and death because they possess the original essence or Qi of life. Unlike other organs, when the kidneys fail life ceases to exists. On the other hand, if the kidneys are firm and the essence is flowing then there is life and longevity.

In his book "Foundations of Chinese Medicine, A Comprehensive Text for Acupuncture and Herbalists," Giovanni Maciocia states "Kidney-Yin (left kidney) is the foundational substance for birth, growth and reproduction where kidney-Yang (right kidney) is the motive force of all physiological processes that transforms Kidney Yin." He goes on to say, "The Kidneys are different from other yin organs because they are the foundation for all the Yin and Yang energies of the body, and also because they are the origin of Water and Fire in the body."[195] When Giovanni says "all Yin and Yang energies," he is referring to building cells, tissues, organs and systems of the body from both right and left kidney energy pasted on from each parent, which develops into genetic material.

The Kidneys are one of the most powerful, if not the most powerful organ in the body. Medical science is always looking at the heart having that power. Kidneys are what TCM refers to as the "Original Qi" (the essence of life), where sperm and eggs develops into a human being. The Kidneys determine whether a woman conceives or not and if the male's sperm is able to impregnate a woman. I refer to Kidneys as the Foundation of Spirit, because both kidneys contribute to the process of gestation and the development of life. Life does not exist without Spirit.

The right Kidney is the fire force (Yang) and the left Kidney provides the water function (Yin). Kidney Essence join forces with Lung Qi to create new life, which is witnessed in the sounds of the bedroom through the sacred chants of groaning, which are kidneys sounds. The heavy intense breathing that take place of inhaling (Kidney) and exhaling (Lungs) in conjunction with the groaning sound promotes the interaction between Spirit and the physical world or between sperm and egg.

In the affairs of the bedroom, together groaning sounds and rhythmic motion bring the couples spiritual Kidney energies into balance and harmony creating a pattern through which new life is introduced to the physical world. Conception of new life occurs when both parents Kidney Essences are in harmony. On the other hand, deficiency of Kidney energy promotes infertility and impotence, which many diabetics experience. In TCM, the Kidneys rules over the reproductive system of conception, birth, maturity, development, life, aging and death. As I have briefly shown kidneys are more important then the heart which Kidneys control (see Nourishing and Controlling chart where Kidney controls the activity of the heart providing fire and water to balance the heart's rythm). Kidney Essence, Qi, Yin and Yang are what maintains our life force, especially diabetics. Many diabetics experience renal (kidney) problems that increase their risk of dialysis and/or renal failure resulting in loss of life. Of all the organs in the body, Kidneys are especially important because when Kidneys fail life is over. Where other organs can be jump started and regenerated. As we know diabetics have a higher rate of Kidney failure then non-diabetics. We have to also look at the relationship between the Kidneys, diabetes and polyuria. Polyuria is promoted due to a weakness of Kidney Qi and Yang (right Kidney energy), or deficient Kidney fire. Kidney fire represents the moving energy and functions of the Kidneys ability to promote the transformation of chemical structures within the Kidneys that filter, reabsorb promoting hormonal activity etc.

In discussing the whole idea of genetics within our bloodline, we are referring to balance levels of Kidney Essence and Kidney Qi. In TCM these elements are known as "Jing or Essence" because they are life's foundational transformation from the Spirit world into the physical world. Physiologically, it refers to our inherited genes from people in our bloodline and what is passed down from generation to generation. Essence/Jing is what determines our constitution and the ability of the body to heal and maintain life. Our constitution dictates our susceptibility to risk of diabetes and other illness.

I would like to spend a moment elaborating on the fact of the Kidney's role in the genetic factor related to diabetes. When a woman is impregnated and moves through the stages of gestation to delivery, she exchanges a great deal of her Essence/Jing (genetic material) with her offspring. Her Kidneys are the sites of Jing, Essences, Yin, and Body Fluids and in conjunction with the liver, which stores blood, all of these substances are transported to the uterus where they nourish the fetus. If for any reason these substances are weak or vacuous, then there will be heat and the heat results in thirst and waste disease promoting diabetes. The weak or vacuity of the yin, blood and body fluid can cause the liver to malfunction resulting in liver stagnation reducing the movement of blood. This liver stagnation can turn into heat consuming the water also resulting in wasting disease (diabetes).[196] On another note, the vacuity of the mother's Qi and fire can compromise gestation including lower back pain, edema, inability to consume different types of food and change in temperament. This is why many women complain of lower back pain during gestation.

The genetic material a mother passes on to her child is the encoding of her and the father's Kidney Essence. A large part of that material is hers, but part of it is from the father as well. If either of the patients Kidneys Essence is weak then the child will have a weak constituent that could spill over to their offspring and affect future generations. This also occurs if a woman has another children within six months to a year of the last delivery. It takes a woman's body at least two years to regenerate from the last child. During that time her body is in the healing phase, where her kidneys are working to replenish their selves in order to maintain her bones, reproductive system, brain and bone marrow (postpartum depression), and the aging process. In this society there is little attention placed on the healing process of a woman after gestation. Anyway, men are no exception to the rule; men lose their Kidney Essences every time they ejaculate. This is why after a man ejaculates he has to sleep or rest before engaging in other activities, especially if he has not taken some sort of enhancement substance. During the time of ejaculation, men give away their Kidney fire and Qi. They can feel the results later in life when fire goes out resulting in impotence. In regards to men with diabetes, Impotence can be a result of yin and essences deficiency drained by the fire of diabetes. Their Kidneys are unable to maintain the balance of fire and water leading to yin not being able to nourish the lower burner (pelvis) and the reproductive organs. This happens to men who are diabetic. Because their Kidney fire is weak they encounter Erectile Dysfunction (ED). Because the Kidney essences rule over the brain marrow, there is a possibly this weakness could cause Alzheimer's-dementia or other mental health issues, head hair loss, hypertension, diabetes, renal failure, growth problems, rapid aging and premature death.

Kidneys are also the sites where hormones are manufactured and balanced. They play a major role in the endocrine system, as a matter of fact the adrenal gland sits atop the kidneys. According to Dr. Hammer, the adrenal mendullary glands function relates to kidney yang (fire of the kidney), who's ability is to provide the other organs with drive and mobility to maintain their own special functions. He also makes it clear that the adrenal cortex resembles kidney yin (water-left kidney) and is responsible for anti-inflammatory and water regulating properties and is related to the pituitary gland (the master endocrine gland), where Kidney yang (fire-right kidney) relates to the thyroid. Another interesting scenario is Kidneys are the focal point when "meno starts pausing" (Menopause) it is a hormonal balance of the Kidneys in relationship with the Liver, Heart and Spleen. Heat flashes and sweats are the result of an imbalance between fire (right Kidney) and water, Essence (left Kidney). It is when the "Tian gui" (Heavenly Water-menstruation) ceases to exist and the water of the Kidneys becomes weak and vacuous. The heat is from the lack of water, causes sweating and when the kidneys rebel against the lungs, the lungs are unable to carry out their function of opening and closing the pores allowing the water to run free. Together they act like a steam valve

I have elaborated on the energy of the Kidneys without discussing its emotional side only because of the vast role they play in maintaining life. The emotional side of the Kidneys has to do with Fear. Fear is the emotion that descends from the kidneys, and anxiety is an emotion that ascends to the heart states Leon Hammer, MD, in his book: Dragon Rises, Red Bird Flies Psychology & Chinese Medicine". [197] Fear moves Qi downward affecting the Bladder and injuring the Kidneys. Dr. Hammer expresses this in his statement "Chronic fear moves from superficial to deep, affecting first the Bladder part of the Tai Yang and then going to the Kidneys, the organ with which the Bladder is most closely related within the Five Phase system, as well as complementary organ in the water phase."[198] When fear injures the Kidneys it moves the body away from its ability to maintain life and can increase the aging process. It reduces a person's ability to promote faith in their life. Many diabetics suffer from depression as a result of fear of not being adequate, not sure of where life is going, not having enough finances, not able to harmonize the ego with the world around them, etc. Recently the Journal of American Medicine published an article on depression having a major relationship with diabetes and in the article they where not sure whether depression caused diabetes or once a person had diabetes they became depressed.

In TCM depression is the emotion of the liver, along with anger, anxiety, frustration, and envy. The Kidneys nourish the Liver and when the kidneys are unable to nourish the Liver, it (Liver) can become stagnated, reducing the circulation of blood through the body, resulting in tingling and numbness and other physiological conditions. As I stated earlier, the eyes are the sensory organ of the liver, many diabetics are challenged with eye issues. Kidney Yin nourishes the fluid of the eyes and maintains the pressure within the eyes. Depression, anger and fear reduces the ability for the Liver and Kidneys to nourish the eyes resulting in glaucoma, cataracts, blindness and other eye conditions.

Fear is the emotion of the Kidneys and fear moves the energy downward suppressing the ability to feel free resulting in other mental conditions such as phobias, low self-esteem, and it also affects cognitive behavior. A person who's kidney yin (water) is deficient can become very brutal to their self and society with no compassion for life with anxiety promoting a deficiency of the Spleen increasing the risk factors of diabetes.

Fear reduces a person's willpower to think clearly when it comes to their health, well-being, judgment or their sense of healing. For instance a diabetic knows they should not eat sweet foods because they will increase blood sugar levels. They indulge any way. They rationalize this by saying they will take their medication and balance the sugar. This is fear of not being able to eat like most people and being left out. On the other hand, it is also a lack of willpower. Both of these attributes are kidney related. When looking at the kidneys from Traditional Chinese prospective you will see there are several dynamics related to fear and its impact on diabetes.

In order to fully understand diabetes and assist in reversing and healing the disease, we have to not only look at the physiological but also the emotional relationship of the person in prospective to the disease.

Bladder

In TCM, the function of the bladder is to store urine, a byproduct of the clear separated fluids from the small intestine. It is a determining factor in polyuria. When the bladder's Qi and fire are deficient, they are unable to process the clear fluids and store it for any length of time without creating frequent urination. The bladder's relationship to the kidney is where it receives waste byproducts from the kidney and excretes waste from the body. When this is unable to occur, the urine can weaken the kidney energy or the bladder can become infected (urinary tract infection).

The emotion of the bladder is jealousy. Jealousy can relate to diabetes, as it is an emotion of holding onto and resentment for someone or something. This causes Qi stagnation, which when affecting the bladder, causes heat and deficiency leading into frequent urination where the bladder is unable to maintain its ability to hold on to urine for any length of time. Jealousy can also increase long-standing grudges. Jealousy not only affects the bladder, but also the gallbladder and small intestine, promoting an inability to make decisions or making changes in one's life. This goes back to what I discussed regarding the large intestine and letting go to make changes and release yourself from that comfort zone. The decision-making process has to do with the gallbladder. The connection of the bladder to the small intestine is in the controlling cycle where the bladder controls the small intestine. The emotions of the bladder controls the emotions of the small intestine promoting clarity on the decisions you make about moving from your comfort zone to work and live without diabetes.

The interconnectiveness of the organs, their network, and emotions aid in either you continuing to be a diabetic or you reversing the illness and living life healthy and free. Even if you say none of these emotions apply to me, you should monitor yourself to make sure you have them in check. You will see your health improve as you change your patterns. When you work to balance your emotions, you begin to work outside of your comfort zone and are able to heal. The emotional comfort zone we build around us is what keeps us ill. You can heal and reverse diabetes. You just have to want to, and do the work needed for it to happen. Always check your emotions. I remember, when we use to give workshops I would place a sign at the door that would say "Check Your Emotions at the Door. So, I say to you to check your emotions so you can live.

Case Studies

"Whenever life is, there is the process of building; different elements are brought together into relations which make of them a living whole, capable of functioning together in harmony."

Virginia Hanson
Gifts of the Lotus

Over the past 25 years of assisting people with improving their health, I have learned a lot about people and their ability to want to heal. I have also come to the understanding that you have some people who think about healing, others who talk about healing, and others who do something to heal. In the two short case studies, you will see people who have done something about healing from diabetes and have been successful. The studies I chose are of those who are very sincere about their health. I will not identify the clients by name.

Study 1

An African American male age 62 who has had diabetes for more than 20 years and who takes three different types of medication. He also complained of tingling and numbness in his feet to the point that it hurt for him to walk. His fasting (morning blood sugar level) was between 110 and 120 with the control of the medication and was not overweight. He is a 6 foot 2 inch slim man. He did little to no exercise and his eating habits consisted of fast and greasy foods. He came to see me because he wanted to change his lifestyle and reduce and/or eliminate the diabetes and the tingling and numbness in his feet. He told me that the issues with his feet has him nervous because he has friends who have had amputations of toes and a person had his leg amputated. His first question to me was, can you save my toes.

After the exam of looking at his tongue, taking his pulses and palpating points on his body I was able to develop a protocol for him, consisting of Di Gui Pi Ren Shen, You Gui Wen and Lui Wei Di Huang Wen. The later two formulas are traditional Chinese formulas for the right (You Gui Wen) and left (Lui Wei Di Huang Wen) kidneys. These two formulas improve the kidney Qi as they tonify the kidneys. He administered 6 capsules of each formula a day from five days each week. He abstained from administering them for two days in order for the herbs not to overpower the body's ability to heal it self. He administered the Di Gui Ren Shen in the same manner only at a separate time of the day. The Di Gui Ren Shen is formulated to assist the panaceas/(spleen in Chinese medicine) to rebalance and tonify.

The protocol also included several micronutrients including 200 mcg of chromium, 400 mg magnesium (for optimum absorption 800 mg calcium, 400 vitamin D3), Alpha-Lipoic Acid for the tingling and numbness and B vitamin complex for the nervous system and to assist in the degrading of carbohydrates. Also to assists in the absorption of vitamin B 6 to address the tingling and numbness. The client visited me once a month for a period of six months on the protocol. After the first month the tingling and numbness began to subside by 45%. Within that month his fasting blood sugar levels decreased to 90 to 100. During the day he would chart his blood sugar and found it decreased by 25%. He could still feel some tingling and numbness.

My protocol starts a diabetic off eating and drinking as much green foods as possible. I had one lady who drank and ate almost nothing but green foods for the first two weeks on the program. She noticed a great difference in her blood sugar levels immediately. She was also taking herbs that are part of the protocol. Green foods are God's wonderful healing foods. Within six months the tingling and numbness had disappeared and the clients physician decreased his medicine by 70% and told him to continue doing what he was doing.

Study 2

The client is a 56 year old African American woman who had elevated blood sugar levels, high cholesterol and was 25 pounds overweight, with a normal blood pressure reading. Her doctor tells her that she is pre-diabetic and that she needed to watch her blood sugar numbers. Her physician also told her if her blood sugar level increased she would prescribe medication for her. This client did not want to take pharmaceuticals and sought assistance in natural methods of reducing her blood sugar levels.

The client is married with two adult children, working in a stressful career that had her traveling a great deal of the time. Because she traveled so much, her eating habits were not always stable. The client usually attended meetings while eating her breakfast, lunch and dinner were the foods are not always the best in nutrients. Her eating did not always consist of nutritional foods that would not increase her blood sugar levels. She says she tries to eat healthy most of the time. She informs me that her fasting blood sugar levels are around 100 to 140 and two hours after she ate her blood levels are still high (180's, 190's).

During our first visit, I had her to change the way she looked at food and presented her with options on how to eat foods that would not increase her blood sugar so high. I also introduced her to methods of using the Glycimic Index to balance her food intake. I suggested she take Di Gui Pi Ren Shen, Lui Wei Di Huang Wen and You Gui Wen. I also suggested she take digestive enzymes, multi-vitamins, 1,600 milligrams of magnesium with 2,400 milligrams of calcium. I also suggested that she take Total Essential Fatty Acids (2,400 milligrams a day) and 200 milligrams of Co Enzyme Q 10. Each of these products she would take for five days each week. The reason was so that her body would begin to work along with the supplement and not take over the process that the body is naturally equip to handle.

I placed her on a three point eating regiment that for the first three weeks of the regiment she ate all types of green vegetables (kale, broccoli, spinach, etc) and incorporated Green Earth food (one of my products) in the morning. The green vegetables were consumed raw and cooked. These foods provided her with vital nutrients and chlorophyll. Chlorophyll as stated before cleanses the body and invigorates cell activity. All other types of foods where reduced or eliminated from her eating habit. This process assisted her digestive tract in rebalancing itself and cleansed her system. It was a difficult task, especially because she traveled so much, but she got through it and felt better and her blood sugar levels decrease dramatically.

After three weeks she began to incorporate other foods such as whole grains (brown rice, cous cous, barley, etc) and some fruits. She did not consume a lot of these grains or fruits during the first week. She would eat only one half of an apple or pear a day in the morning after she consumed a half bowl of oatmeal with no sugar or milk. The second week she increased her intake of these foods and at the same time continued to consume green vegetables. Her slow integration of grains and fruits allowed her to maintain a fasting blood sugar level of 80-95 and two hours after eating her blood sugar level was in the 120's and 130's. Within three weeks of introducing whole grains and fruits back into her eating habit, they went from small portions to a full meal. At the end of three weeks she was consuming at least one piece of fruit a day and every other day some type of whole grain.

During the third phase of the program she incorporated fish, and chicken into her eating habit over a period of three weeks. She started off with small portions and as the weeks went on she increased her portions to a full meal. These products where baked, broiled, stewed or grilled. She only consumed cold-water and white meat fish (salmon, whiting, haddock, etc.) and no shellfish. She only ate the breast of the chicken and the chickens were free range. The breast of a chicken is vein less and has good quality protein.

After the third phase of the regiment she incorporated read meat back into her eating habit, however, she only consumed one-half ounce per meal. She only consumed red meat twice a week in the form of lamb. Through the regiment she no longer drank and ate at the same time and combines her foods well. The client has loss 32 pounds since the time she started the program in 2008. At her last medical check up her HC1a was 5 and her cholesterol was in the 150 range, where before it was over 230. She is still eating in the way I showed her and is feeling good.

These are just two of the many successes that have happened from lifestyle changes and using natural products. Diabetes can be reversed. It is about what you do to reverse it and how you stay the course. It is the course that matters.

QI Gong (Physical Activity)

Studies have shown there is a need for exercise within the entire country, especially amongst overweight and obese people who are at great risk for type 2 diabetes. Physical activity assists in the promotion of blood circulation, reduction in adiposity, and decrease in cholesterol and has been known to aid diabetics in eliminating diabetic's medication.[199]

Exercise promotes the uptake of glucose into the cells by GLUT-4 transporters, which is the same method used by insulin.

When a diabetic develops a consistent exercise program they begin to see a body reshaped and find they have more energy. A good exercise program is preformed at list three times a week for 30 minutes to an hour per session. The exercise does not have to be heavy or vigorous, but steady and consistent. Some diabetics chose to run which is acceptable they have to run on a surface that is gentle on their knees. In this case treadmill, grass, a track, or Astro turf are good surfaces to run on. Yoga, Tai Chi, and Qi Gong, which are Eastern exercises that many people in the United States have adopted. These are good exercise programs for diabetics. They are very stimulating workouts promoting cardiovascular activity and are very gentle, soft, flowing and not only increases the circulation of blood. They also stretch the muscle to a point where they become relaxed and energized. These exercises not only increase glucose uptake, but they also reduce other health conditions.

Conclusion

The Desire to Heal Begins with You Loving You(TM)
Dr. Akmal Muwwakkil

Within this book there is information that provides proof that type 1 and type 2 diabetes mellitus are far from being a genetically determined disease. It reveals facts that diabetes is a disease of the digestive tract reducing the body from digesting, absorbing, and assimilating nutrients resulting in both types of diabetes. It is shown in several cases when micronutrients are properly administered the prevalence of diabetes risk declines. On the other hand, when diabetics increase their intake of micronutrients their elevated glucose levels reduce and in some cases their blood sugar levels become in the normal range eliminating the need for pharmacological substance. The increase of micronutrients supplementation also has an effect on the many complications and other disease related to diabetes.

The study concludes that when people consume foods with good nutritional values, exercise consistently and use nutritional supplementations, their risk of diabetes is reduced. Diabetics are able to reduce and/or eliminate their medications. It also shows where mothers have to maintain a level of wellness and breastfeed their children in order to reduce the prevalence of type 1 diabetes, warding off viruses and increasing immunity and building gut flora of their children. In order to reduce the increase of type 2 diabetes amongst children and adolescents families have to prepare meals at home and eat out less so their children receive good quality food with vital nutrients to increase their health and well being.

There is a growing need to establish a good relationship between wholistic health therapists who work in the field of diabetes and medical physicians. There is an urgent need to combine research and use of micronutrients and phytonutrients to eradicate the prevalence of diabetes.

References

1. Campbell, C.T., PhD, Campbell II, T.M.: Problems We Face Solutions We Need; The China Study Startling Impalications For Diet, Weight Loss and Long-Term Health: Benbella Books, Inc, 6440 N. Central Expressway, suite 617, Dallas, TX 75206: PP15
2. Bryan, C.P, AAA Disease: The Papyrus Ebers Oldest Medical Book in The World: The African Islamic Mission Publications, New York, NY
3. Flaws. B, Kuchinski.L, Casanas.R, MD: The Treatment of Diabetes Mellitus with Chinese Medicine: Blue Poppy Press' A division of Blue Poppy Enterprises, Inc: 5441 Western Ave., Suite 2, Boulder, CO 80301
4. Flaws. B, Kuchinski.L, Casanas.R, MD: The Treatment of Diabetes Mellitus with Chinese Medicine: Blue Poppy Press' A division of Blue Poppy Enterprises, Inc: 5441 Western Ave., Suite 2, Boulder, CO 80301
5. The History of Diabetes: Canadian Diabetes Association Website: ww.diabetes.ca/Section About/timelie.asp
6. Flaws. B, Kuchinski.L, Casanas.R, MD: The Treatment of Diabetes Mellitus with Chinese Medicine: Blue Poppy Press' A division of Blue Poppy Enterprises, Inc: 5441 Western Ave., Suite 2, Boulder, CO 80301
7. The History of Diabetes: Canadian Diabetes Association Website: ww.diabetes.ca/Section About/timelie.asp
8. Flaws. B, Kuchinski.L, Casanas.R, MD: The Treatment of Diabetes Mellitus with Chinese Medicine: Blue Poppy Press' A division of Blue Poppy Enterprises, Inc: 5441 Western Ave., Suite 2, Boulder, CO 80301:PP 2
9. Flaws, B. Kuchinski, L. Casanas, R, M.D.: Diabetes Mellitus & western Medicine: The Treatment of Diabetes Mellitus with Chinese Medicine; A Textbook and Clinical Manual: Blue Poppy Press A Division of Blue Poppy Enterprise, Inc, 5441 Western Ave., Suite 2, Boulder, CO 80301: PP3

10. Flaws, B. Kuchinski, L. Casanas, R, M.D.: Diabetes Mellitus & Western Medicine: The Treatment of Diabetes Mellitus with Chinese Medicine; A Textbook and Clinical Manual: Blue Poppy Press A Division of Blue Poppy Enterprise, Inc, 5441 Western Ave., Suite 2, Boulder, CO 80301: PP3
11. National Diabetes Statistic, National Diabetes Information Clearinghouse (NDIC): Service of the National Institute of Diabetes, and Digestive and Kidney Disease (NIDDK), NIH; 1 Information Way, Bethesda, MD 20892
12. (Amylin Pharmaceuticals, inc and Eli Lilly and CDC national Estimates on Diabetes)
13. 3. National Diabetes education program
14. National Institute of Diabetes and Digestive Diseases, National Diabetes Statistics Fact Sheet: General Information and National Estimate on Diabetes in the United States, 2005. Bethesda, MD; U.S. Department of Health and Human Services, National Institute of Health.
15. *King H, Aubert RE, Herman WH*
16. Marion J, Anti-Aging Manual, The Encyclopedia of Natural Health; Conditions & Cures; Diabetes 764
17. National Diabetes Statistics; National Diabetes Information Clearinghouse (NDIC): National Institute of Diabetes and Digestive and Kidney Disease (NIDDK), NIH; 1 Information Way, Bethesda, MD 20892-3560
18. Diabetes Statistics: American Diabetes Association; 1701 North Beauregard Street, Alexandria, VA 22311
19. CDC National Diabetes Fact Sheet 2005
20. prevent and treat diabetes with natural medicine pp 62
21. Curtis J. Et Al, Gerstein, RB Haynes, Eds: Diagnosis and Short-Term Clinical consequences of Diabetes In Children and adolescents In HC: Evidence Based Diabetes Care: Hamilton, On: BC Decker, PP107-123
22. Dana Dabelea, MD, PhD. Lead Investigator: An Epidemic of Type 2 Diabetes in Youth: Department of Preventive Medicine and Biometrico, University of Colorado School of Medicine.
23. Whitaker, J. MD, What to Expect If You Have Diabetes, Reversing Diabetes PP9
24. Murray, Michael, ND. A Closer Look at Risk Factors for Type 1 Diabetes: How to Prevent and Treat Diabetes with Natural Medicine; PP29-30
25. Hyoty H. Enterovirus infections and type 1 diabetes. Ann Med. 2002;34:138-147
26. Murray Michael, ND. A Closer Look at Risk Factors for Type 1 Diabetes: How to Prevent and Treat Diabetes with Natural Medicine; PP 39

27. Murry Michael, ND: A Closer Look at Risk factors for Type 1 Diabetes; How to Prevent and treat diabetes with Natural Medicine: Riverhead Book, The Berkley Publishing Group, 375 Hudson street, New York, NY 10014;PP 37
28. Murray Michael, N.D., A Closer Look at Risk Factors for Type 1 Diabetes: How to Prevent and Treat Diabetes with Natural Medicine: The Berkley Publishing Group, 375 Hudson Street, New York, NY: PP37
29. Murray Michael, N.D., A Closer Look at Risk Factors for Type 1 Diabetes
30. Murray Michael, N.D., A Closer Look at Risk Factors for Type 1 Diabetes
31. MilkSucks.com: Georgetown University School of Medicine, 1994; Annals of Allergy
32. Murray Frank; Natural Supplements for Diabetes pp 79
33. Murray Michael, N.D. How to Prevent and Treat Diabetes with Natural Medicine PP45
34. Murray Michael N.D. How to Prevent and treat Diabetes with Natural Medicine PP37
35. Murray, M, ND, A Closer Look at Risk Factors for Type 2 Diabetes, How to Prevent and Treat Diabetes with Natural Medicine: The Berkley publishing Group, 375 Hundson Street, New York, NY 10014: PP 66-67
36. Hu BF, MD, Dietary Patterns and Risk for Type 2 Diabetes Mellitus in Men, Annals of Internal Medicine Feb 2002;vol 136 issue 3;201-9
37. Murray, M ND, How to prevent and Treat Diabetes with Natural: The Berkley publishing Group, 375 Hundson Street, New York, NY 10014: pp63
38. Otto Tschritter, Andreas Fritsche, Claus Thamer, Michael Haap, Fatemeh Shirkavand, Stefanie Rahe, Harald staiger, Elke Maerker, Hans Haring and Michael Stumvoll from the Medizinische Klinik, Abteilung fur Endokrinologie, Stoffwechsel und Pathobiochemine, Eberhard-Karls-Universitat, Tubingen, Germany Plasma Adiponectin Concentrations Predict Insulin Sensitivity of Both Glucose and Lipid Metabaolism Diabetes, vol 52; Feb 2003.
39. Center for Disease Control and Prevention; Overweight and Obesity: Website: www.cdc.gov/nccdphp/dnpa/obesity/trend/maps.
40. Critser Greg: Who Let the Calories In; Fat Land: Houghton Mifflin Company; 215 Park Avenue South, New York, NY 10003:PP 32
41. United States Department of Agriculture: USDA Finds More and More American Eat Out, offers for making Healthier Food Choices: www.ars.usda.gov/is/pr/1996/eatout1196.htm?pf=1

42. Al Rosenbloom, Jr Joe, RS Young, WE Winter: Children's Medical Service Center, University of Florida College of Medicine, Gainsville, Fl 32608, USA: Emerging Epidemic of Type 2 Diabetes in Youth: Diabetes Care; vol 22, iss 2 PP 345-54

43. Critser Greg: What Fat Is, What Fat Isn't ; Fat Land: Houghton Mifflin Company; 215 Park Avenue South, New York, NY 10003:PP 111

44. Lee Lita, PhD, Tuner, Lisa, Burton Goldberg: Diabetes; The Enzyme Cure; How Plant Enzymes Can Help You Relieve 36 Health Problems: Future Medicine Publicating1640 Tiburon, Ca 94920: PP123

45. Frank Murray; Natural Supplements for Diabetes Reduce Your Risk and Lower Insulin Dependency with Natural Remedies: The Complications of Cardiovascular Disease: Hampton Road Publishing Company, Inc. 1125 Stoney Ridge Road, Charlottesville, VA 22902: PP42

46. Frank Murray; Natural Supplements for Diabetes Reduce Your Risk and Lower Insulin Dependency with Natural Remedies: The Complications of Cardiovascular Disease: Hampton Road Publishing Company, Inc. 1125 Stony Ridge Road, Charlottesville, VA 22902: PP40

47. de Munter JS, Hu FB, Spiegelman D, Franz M, van Dam RM; Whole grain, bran, and germ intake and risk of type 2 diabetes: a prospective cohort study and systematic review. Plos Med. 2007; 4:e261.

48. Whole Grains The Inside Story: Nutrition Action Health letter: Center for Science in the Public Interest, 1875 Connecticut Ave, N.W. Washington, D.C. 20009PP 3- 5

49. Murray, M. a close Look at risk Factors for Type 2 Diabetes; Eating the wrong Types of Fats: How to Prevent and Treat Diabetes with Natural Medicine: PP84

50. Whitker, J. M.D., The Diabetic Diet: Where Do Protein and Fat Fit In: Reversing Diabetes: Time Waner Book group, 1271 Avenue of the Americas, New York, NY 10020:PP 136-37

51. Lopez, D.A. M.D., Williams, R.M., M.D., Ph.D, Miehlke, K, M.D.: Introduction; Enzymes The Fountain of Life: The Neville Press, Inc, 18 Broad Street, suite 601, Charleston, SC 29401:PP1

52. Cahokia, A.J., D.C., Jump Start Digestion, Enzymes & Enzyme Therapy; How to Jump Start your way to Lifelong Good Health: Keats Publishing, Inc, 27 Pine street, Box 876, New Canaan, Connecticut 06840: PP 23

53. Lopez, D.A. M.D., Williams, R.M., M.D., PhD, Miehlke, K, M.D.: Introduction; Enzymes The Fountain of Life: The Neville Press, Inc, 18 Broad Street, suite 601, Charleston, SC 29401:PP108

54   Lopez, D.A. M.D., Williams, R.M., M.D., PhD, Miehlke, K, M.D.: Introduction; Enzymes The Fountain of Life: The Neville Press, Inc, 18 Broad Street, suite 601, Charleston, SC 29401:PP 9-10
55   (5. Dr. James E. Everhart: Epidemiology and Clinical Trials Branch, Division of Digestive Diseases and Nutrition, National Institute of Diabetes and Digestive and Kidney Diseases, NIH).
56   Murray, F. Chromium; Natural Supplement for Diabetes Reduce Your Risk and Lower Your Insulin Dependency with Natural Remedies: Hampton Roads Publishing Company, 1125 Stony Ridge Road, Charlottesville, VA 22902: PP286
57   Everheart, E. James, MD, MPH: Chapter 21, Digestive Disease and Diabetes: NIH National Diabetes Information Clearing House: National Institute of diabetes and Digestive and Kidney Disease: NIDDK, NIH Building 31, room 9a06, 31 Center Driver, MSC 2560, Bethesda, MD 20892-2560, USA
58   Everheart, E. James, MD, MPH: Chapter 21, Digestive Disease and Diabetes: NIH national Diabetes Information Clearing House: National Institute of Diabetes and Digestive and Kidney Disease: NIDDK, NIH Building 31, room 9a06, 31 Center Driver, MSC 2560, Bethesda, MD 20892-2560, USA
59   Watson, B N.D., Smith, L, M.D., Leaky Gut Syndrome: Gut Solutions Natural Solution To Your Digestive Problems; Renew Life Press and Information Services, 2076 Sunnydale Drive Clearwater, Fl 33765: PP153
60   Whitaker, J, M.D., A Diet to Improve Insulin Sensitivity: Reversing Diabetes; reducing or Even Eliminating Your Dependence On Insulin or Oral Drugs: Time Warner Book Group, 1271 Avenue of the Americas, New York, NY 10020: PP 107
61   Whitaker, J, M.D., A Diet to Improve Insulin Sensitivity: Reversing Diabetes; Reducing or Even Eliminating Your Dependence On Insulin or Oral Drugs: Time Warner Book Group, 1271 Avenue of the Americas, New York, NY 10020: PP 107
62   Casper, D., MA, Stone T., ND, CN: Processed Food; Modern Foods: The Sabotage of Earths Food Supply: Center Point Press, PMB 143, 12463 Rancho Bernardo Road, San Diego, CA 92128
63   The Merck Manual of Medical Information Second Home Edition: Pocket Books: Simon & Schuster;1230 Avenue of the Americas, New York, NY10020: PP920

64. Drexel H, M.D., Marte T, M.D., Langer P, and PhD, Saely H. C, M.D.: Is Atherosclerosis in Diabetes and Impaired Fasting Glucose Divern by Elevated LDL Cholesterol by Decreased HDL Cholesterol? : Diabetic Care28:101-107,2005
65. The Institute of Functional Medicine: Fats: Clinical Nutrition A Functional Medicine Approach, second edition: The Functional Medicine P.O. Box 1697 Gig Harbor, Washington, 98335, USA: PP70
66. The Institute of Functional Medicine: Fats: Clinical Nutrition A Functional Medicine Approach, second edition: The Functional Medicine P.O. Box 1697 Gig Harbor, Washington, 98335, USA: PP70
67. Wildman,R,PhD,RD. Fats and Cholesterol are not all bad: The Nutritionist; food, Nutrition, and Optimal Heath: The Haworth Press, Inc 10 Alice Street, Binghamton, NY 13904-1580:PP119
68. Balch, P, CNC, Balch J., M.D., Lecithin: Prescription for Nutritional Healing Third Edition; Penguin Putnam Inc 375 Hudson Street, New York, NY 10014:PP 74
69. Balch, P, CNC, Balch J., M.D., Lecithin: Prescription for Nutritional Healing Third Edition; Penguin Putnam Inc 375 Hudson Street, New York, NY 10014:PP 74
70. Albion Research Notes; Mineral Considerations in Diabetes Mellitus: Albion Research Notes; Albion Advanced Nutrition, Inc, 101 North Main Street, Clearfield, Utah, 84015:June 2002, vol 11 (2)
71. Mineral Considerations in Diabetes Mellitus: Albion Research Notes, A Compilation of Vital Research Update on Human Nutrition; June 2002; vol 11(2): Albion advanced Nutrition, P.O. Box 750, Clearfield, Utah 84089
72. Mineral Considerations in Diabetes Mellitus: Albion Research Notes, A Compilation of Vital Research Update on Human Nutrition; June 2002; vol 11(2): Albion advanced Nutrition, P.O. Box 750, Clearfield, Utah 84089
73. Murray, M ND, Pizzonrno, J., ND, Encyclopedia of Natural Medicine, 417
74. Murray, M, ND, Diet Therapy in Managing Diabetes, How to Prevent and Treat Diabetes with Natural Medicine: The Berkley Publishing Group, 375 Hudson Street, New York, NY10014: PP155
75. Murray, F, Chromium, Natural Supplements for Diabetes, 282
76. Anderson Richard A. PhD. Nutritional Factors influencing the Glucose/insulin system: Chromium, Journal of the American College of Nutrition, vol16 (5):404-410, 1997

77 Balch, P, CNC, Blach, J, M.D., Chromium; Prescription for Nutritional Healing, Third Edition: Penguin Putnam, Inc, 375 Hudson Street, New York, NY 10014: PP 27
78 Murray, M, ND, Pizzorno, J, ND; Encyclopedia of Natural medicine: Magnesium 420-21
79 Frank M: Magnesium; Natural Supplements for Diabetes: Hampton Roads Publishing Company, Inc, 1125 Stony Ridge Road, Charlottesville, VA 22902:PP 41-2
80 Takaya, J, Higashino, H, Kobayashi, Y, Intercellular Magnesium and Insulin Resistance, Magnesium Research;vol17 (2):126-36 June 2004
81 Lepore, D. ND, Magnesium, The Ultimate Healing System:
82 Lepore, D ND, The Ultimate Healing System; Lecithin: 131-2
83 Balch J, MD, Stengler, M, ND; Prescription for Natural Cures: Diabetes 193
84 Hamilton, Kirk. "Diabetes Mellitus and Vitamin B6," The expert Speak. Sacramento, Calif.: I.T. service, 1996, PP 102-103 Murray, Also Mohan, Chandra, Ph.D. "Vitamin B6 Metabolism and Diabetes," Biochemical and Metabolic Biology 52: 10-17, 1994
85 Julie c. Will, Earls Ford, Barbara A. Bowman, The Division of Nutrition and Physical Activity, National Center for Chronic Disease Prevention, Center for Disease Control and Prevention, Atlanta, GA: Serum vitamin C concentrations and Diabetes: finding from the Third National Health and Nutrition examination survey, 1988-1994.
86 Murray, Michael, ND. Diabetic Complications: An Overview: Nutrient Deficiency: How to Prevent and Treat Diabetes with Natural Medicine: The Berkley Publishing Group, New York, NY. 2003, PP 239
87 Lepore, Donald, ND. B 12; The Ultimate Healing System: The Illustrated Guide To Muscle Testing & Nutrition: Woodland Publishing, Inc. PP 28
88 Will, Julie C., Ford Earl S., Bowman, Barbara A, Serum Vitamin C Concentrations and Diabetes: Finding from the Third National Health and Nutrition Examination Survey 1988-1994. Published: American Journal of Clinical Nutrition: vol 70, 1999, PP49-52
89 Murray, Michael, ND. Diet Therapy in Managing Diabetes: How to Prevent and Treat Diabetes with Natural Medicine: The Berkley Publishing Group, 375 Hudson Street, New York, NY. 2003, PP 156
90 , Michael, ND. Diet Therapy in Managing Diabetes: How to Prevent and Treat Diabetes with Natural Medicine: The Berkley Publishing Group, 375 Hudson Street, New York, NY. 2003, PP 157

91. Murray, Frank. Natural Supplements for Diabetes; Vitamin C: Pfleger, R. and colleagues, University of Vienna, 258
92. Vitamin E and Cardiovascular Protection in Diabetes: Antioxidants May Offer Particular Advantage in This High Risk Group: British Medical Journal:314;1845-1846, June 28, 1997
93. Murray Frank, Vitamin E; Natural Supplements for Diabetes: reduce your Risk and Lower Your Insulin Dependency with Natural Remedies, Hampton Roads Publishing Company, Inc, 1125 Stony Ridge Road, Charlottesville, VA 22902: PP 272
94. Whitaker, Julian, M.D. Nutritional Supplements for Diabetes: Reversing Diabetes, Reducing or Even Elimination Your Dependence on Insulin or Oral Drugs. New York, NY, Time Warner Book Group, 1987, pp 180
95. Frank Murray, Vitamin E: Natural Supplement for Diabetes, Reduce Your Risk and Lower Your Insulin Dependency with Natural Remedies. Charlottesville, VA, Hampton Roads Publishing Company, Inc, 2003, PP 273
96. Frank Murray, Selenium: Natural Supplement for Diabetes, Reduce Your Risk and Lower Your Insulin Dependency with Natural Remedies. Charlottesville, VA, Hampton Roads Publishing Company, Inc, 2003, PP 298
97. Murray Michael, N.D. Pizzorno Joseph, N.D., Niacin and Niacinamide: Encyclopedia of Natural Medicine. New York, NY, Three River Press, 1997, PP418-9
98. Frank Murray, Niacin; The B-Complex Vitamins: Natural Supplements for Diabetes Reduce Your Risk and Lower Your Insulin Dependency with Natural Remedies. Charlottesville, VA, Hampton Roads Publishing Company, Inc. 2003 PP 232
99. Murray Michael, N.D. Pizzorno Joseph, N.D., Niacin and Niacinamide: Encyclopedia of Natural Medicine. New York, NY, Three River Press, 1997, PP418-9
100. Murry Michael, N.D. Lyon, Michael, M.D. Natural Products for Type 1 Diabetes: How to Prevent and treat Diabetes with Natural Medicine. New York, NY, The Berkley Publishing Group, 2003, PP 178
101. Koutsikos D. Forutounas C; Kapetanaki A; Agroyannis B; TzanatosA H; Rammos G; Kopelias I; Bosiolis B; Bovoleti O; Darema M; Sallum G: Oral Glucose Tolerance Test After High-Doses I.V. Biotin Administration in Normoglucemic Hemodialysis Patients: Ren Fail, 1996 Jan, 18:1, 131-7
102. Murry Michael, N.D. Lyon, Michael, M.D. Natural Products for Type 1 Diabetes: How to Prevent and treat Diabetes with Natural Medicine. New York, NY, The Berkley Publishing Group, 2003, PP 178

103. Frank Murray, The B-Complex Vitamins: Natural Supplements for Diabetes Reduce Your Risk and Lower Your Insulin Dependency with Natural Remedies. Charlottesville, VA, Hampton Roads Publishing Company, Inc. 2003 PP 251
104. Frank Murray, The B-Complex Vitamins: Natural Supplements for Diabetes Reduce Your Risk and Lower Your Insulin Dependency with Natural Remedies. Charlottesville, VA, Hampton Roads Publishing Company, Inc. 2003 PP 251
105. Whitaker, Julian, M.D. Natural Supplements for Diabetes Reversing Diabetes Reduce or Even Eliminate Your Dependence on Insulin or Oral Drugs. New York, NY, Time Warner Book Group, 1987, PP 170
106. Whitaker, Julian, M.D. Natural Supplements for Diabetes Reversing Diabetes Reduce or Even Eliminate Your Dependence on Insulin or Oral Drugs. New York, NY, Time Warner Book Group, 1987, PP 170
107. Whitaker, Julian, M.D. Natural Supplements for Diabetes Reversing Diabetes Reduce or Even Eliminate Your Dependence on Insulin or Oral Drugs. New York, NY, Time Warner Book Group, 1987, PP 171
108. Frank Murray, Vanadium: Natural Supplements for Diabetes Reduce Your Risk and Lower Your Insulin Dependency with Natural Remedies. Charlottesville, VA, Hampton Roads Publishing Company, Inc. 2003 PP 301
109. Frank Murray, Vanadium: Natural Supplements for Diabetes Reduce Your Risk and Lower Your Insulin Dependency with Natural Remedies. Charlottesville, VA, Hampton Roads Publishing Company, Inc. 2003 PP 303
110. Murray Frank, Zinc, Diet Therapy in Managing Diabetes: Natural Supplements for Diabetes Reduce Your Risk and Lower Your Insulin Dependency with Natural Remedies. Charlottesville, VA, Hampton Road Publishing Company, Inc 2003: PP 161
111. Frank Murray, Zinc: Natural Supplements for Diabetes Reduce Your Risk and Lower Your Insulin Dependency with Natural Remedies. Charlottesville, VA, Hampton Roads Publishing Company, Inc. 2003 PP 306
112. Murray Frank, Vitamin D: Natural Supplements for Diabetes Reduce Your Risk and Lower Your Insulin Dependency with Natural Remedies. Charlottesville, VA, Hampton Road Publishing Company, Inc 2003: PP 267-68
113. Frank Murray, Why You Need to Exercise to Reduce Your Diabetes Risk: Natural Supplements for Diabetes, Reduce Your Risk and Lower

	Your Insulin Dependency with Natural Remedies. Charlottesville, VA, Hampton Roads Publishing Company, Inc. 2003 PP 175
114	Frank Murray, Why You Need to Exercise to Reduce Your Diabetes Risk: Natural Supplements for Diabetes, Reduce Your Risk and Lower Your Insulin Dependency with Natural Remedies. Charlottesville, VA, Hampton Roads Publishing Company, Inc. 2003 PP 177
115	Malhotra, V., S. Singh, O.P. Tandon, S.V. Madhu, A. Prasad, and S.B. Sharma: Study of Yoga Asanas in assessment of Pulmonary Function in NIDM Patients: Indian Journal of Physiology and Pharmacology, July 202, 46(3):313-320. PMID
116	Center for Disease Control and Prevetion
117	Murray, M. N.D., Diabetes Complications: An Overview: How to Prevent and Treat Dibetes with Natural Medicine: Riverhead Books The Berkley Publishing Group 375 Hudson Street, New York, NY 10014: PP 239
118	Raghuveer, G., Effects of Vitamin E on resistance Vessels Endothelial Dysfunction Induced by Methionine, American Journal of Cardiology, 88:285-290, 2001
119	Braverman, E. M.D., Homocysteine; The Predictor of Heart Disease: The Healing Nutrients Within New Third Edition: Basic Health Pubblication, Inc 8200 Boulevard East, North Bergen, NJ 07047
120	Fran Murray, Homocysteine: More Dangerous than Cholesterol?: Natural Supplements For Diabetes, Reduce Your Risk and Lower Your Insulin Dependency with Natural Remedies: Hampton Roads Publishing Company, Inc, 1125 Stoney Ridge Road, Charlottsville, VA 22902: PP 131
121	Marion, J, B; High Blood Pressure, Conditions & Cures: The Encyclopedia of natural Health: Information Pioneer Publ., P.O. Box 7, South Woodstock, Connecticut 06267: PP 685
122	Marion, J, B; High Blood Pressure, Conditions & Cures: The Encyclopedia of natural Health: Information Pioneer Publ., P.O. Box 7, South Woodstock, Connecticut 06267: PP 685
123	Statistics Related to Overweight and Obesity; National Institute of Diabetes and Digestive and Kidney Diseases: 1 Win Way, Bethesda, MD 20892-3665
124	Prevalence of Overweight Among Children and Adolescents: United States, 1999-2002: US Department of Health and Human Services; Center for Disease Control and Prevention; National Center for Health Statistics: Hyattsville, MD 20782

125. Healthy Youth ; Childhood Obesity: Center for Disease Control and Prevention; 1600 Cliton Road, Atlanta, GA 30333 USA
126. Cherewatenko, V, M.D.: Diabetes Disease Review: The Diabetes Cure: HarperCollins Publishing Inc., 10 East 53rd Street, New York, NY 10022: PP 221
127. Ellis, J. M., M.D., and Pamplin, J.,: Vitamin B6 Therapy: Avery Publishing Group, New York: PP 69
128. Murray, M, N.D., Recommendations for Specific Chronic Complications: How to Prevent and Treat Diabetes with Natural Medicine: Riverhead Books; The Berkley Publishing Grooup 375 Hudson Street, New York, NY 10014: 266
129. Murray, F., The B-Complex Vitamin: Natural Supplements for Diabetes: Hampton Roads Publishing Company, Inc. 1125 Stoney Ridge Road, Charlottesville, VA 22902: PP 239
130. Murray, F., The B-Complex Vitamin: Natural Supplements for Diabetes: Hampton Roads Publishing Company, Inc. 1125 Stoney Ridge Road, Charlottesville, VA 22902: PP 338
131. Abuaisha B.B., Acupuncture for the Treatment of Chronic Painful Diabetes Neuropathy: A Long Term Study: Diabetes Research and Clinical Practice:39:115-121,1998
132. Rains C, Bryson HM. Topical Capsaicin. A Review of TS Pharmacological Properties and Therapeutic Potential in Post-Herpetic Neuralgia, Diabetic Neuropathy and Osteoarthritis: Drug Aging; 1995;7:317-328
133. Diabetes-Inducted Change in lens antioxidant Status, Glucose Utilization and Energy Metabolisms Effect of Dl-Alpha-Lipoic Acid: Diabetiologia 41:1442-50, 1988
134. Jaques, P. F., and L. T. Chylack Jr 1991. Epidemiologic Evidence of a Role for the Antioxidant Vitamins and Caroteniods in Cataract Prevention. American Journal of Clinical Nutrition 53:352S-55S. (Knekt, P., M. Heliovaara, A. Rissanen et, al. 192. Serum Antioxidant Vitamins and Risk of Cataract. British Medical Jouranl 305:1392-94.) (Mares-Perlman, J. A., et al 2000. Vitamin supplement use and incident cataracts I a population-based study. Archives of Ophthalmology 118:1556-63
135. Knekt, P., M. Heliovaara, A. Rissanen et, al. 192. Serum Antioxidant Vitamins and Risk of Cataract. British Medical Jouranl 305:1392-94.
136. Mares-Perlman, J. A., et al 2000. Vitamin Supplement Use and Incident of Cataracts I A Populated-based Study. Archives of Ophthalmology 118:1556-63

137 Ludwig, D. Dietary Glycemic Index and Obesity: J. Nutrition 2000: 130:280S -3S
138 Ludwig D, Majzoub J. Al-Zahrani A, Dallal G, Blanco I, Roberts S.: High Glycemic Index Foods, Overeating, and Obesity: Pediatrics [serial online] 1999; 103:e 26 internet: *http://www.pediatrics.org/cgi/content/full/103/3/e36* (accessed 9 April 2002)
139 Frances Chi S. Dal Ml, Augustine L, et al. Dietary Glycemic Load and Colorectal Cancer Risk> Ann Oncol 2001; 12:173-8
140 Augustine L. Dietary Glycemic Index and Glycemic Load in Breast Cancer Risk: A Case Control Study. Annoncol (inpress)
141 Luis, Willett W, Stumper M, et al. A Perspective Study of Dietary Glycemic Load, Carbohydrate Intake and Risk of Coronary Heart Disease in US Women. Am J Clin Nutrition 2000;71:1455-61
142 Goettemoeller J: Research Review: Stavis Sweet Recipes: Vital Health Publishing, P.O. Box 544, Bloomingdale, Il 60108:PP 11-12
143 Pitchford, P. Sweeteners: Healing With Whole Foods Oriental Traditions and Modern Nutrition: North Atlantic Books P.O. Box 12327, Berkeley, CA 94701:PP 154
144 Murray, M, ND., Beutler, J, RRT, RCP,: Understanding The Terminology; Understanding Fats & Oils Your Guide to Healing with Essential Fatty Acids: Progressive Health Publishing 315 First Street #U-198, Encinitas, CA 92024: PP 2
145 Murray, M, ND., Beutler, J, RRT, RCP,: Understanding The Terminology; Understanding Fats & Oils Your Guide to Healing with Essential Fatty Acids: Progressive Health Publishing 315 First Street #U-198, Encinitas, CA 92024: PP 17
146 Champe, P.C, Harvey, A. R.; Metabolism of Dietary lipids: Biochemistry 2nd edition: Lippincott Williams & Wilkins 530 Walnut Street, Philadelphia, PA 19106
147 Murray, M, ND., Beutler, J, RRT, RCP,: Understanding The Terminology; Understanding Fats & Oils Your Guide to Healing with Essential Fatty Acids: Progressive Health Publishing 315 First Street #U-198, Encinitas, CA 92024: PP 10-11
148 Wikipedia The Free Encyclopedia: http:///.en.wikipedia.org/wiki/lipid_peroxidation
149 American Heart Association: http://www.americanheart.org/presenter.jhtml?identifier=3045792

150 Marion, J, Unsaturated Fatty Acids (EFAs), Anti-Aging Manual: Information Pioneers Publ., P.O. Box 7, South Woodstock, Connecticut 06267: PP 90

151 Murray, T. M., ND, Beutler, J. R.R.T., R.C.P.: Cell Membrane Alteration and Disease: Understanding Fats & Oils Your Guide To Healing With Essential Fatty Acids; Progressive Health Publishing; 315 first Street #U-198, Encinitas, CA 92024PP17

152 Murray, T. M., ND, Beutler, J. R.R.T., R.C.P.: Cell Membrane Alteration and Disease: Understanding fats & Oils Your Guide To Healing With Essential Fatty Acids; Progressive Health Publishing; 315 First Street #U-198, Encinitas, CA 92024: PP17

153 Hamdorf, G, M.D. Thioctic Acid A Rational Remedy for the Treatment of Diabetic Polyneuropathy, Experimental Clinical Endocrinology and Diabetes 104:126-127, 1995

154 Packer, Lester, PhD; Alpha-Lipoic Acid as a Biological Antioxidant free Radical Biology and Medicine 19 (2): 227-250, 1995)

155 Murray, F, Alpha-Lipoic Acid: Natural Supplements for Diabetes: Hampton Roads Publishing Company, Inc. 1125 Stoney Ridge Road, Charlottesville, VA 22902:317

156 Balch P, A. CNC, Balch F. M.D.: Lecithin: Prescription for Nutritional Healing Third Edition: Penguin Putnam Inc. 375 Hudson Street, New York, NY 10014:pp74-75

157 Murray, M. ND, Pizzorno, J., ND: Diabetes Mellitus; Encyclopedia of Natural Medicine: Three River Press, New York, NY PP 419

158 Murray, M, ND.: Vitamin C; Encyclopedia of Nutritional Supplements: Prima Publishing, P.O. Box 11260BK, Rocklin, CA 9567: PP 62

159 Murray, M, ND. :Vitamin C: Encyclopedia of Nutritional Supplements: Prima Publishing, P.O. Box 11260BK, Rocklin, CA 9567: PP 59

160 Lepore, D, N.D.: Vitamin E; The Ultimate Healing System The Illustrated Guide to Muscle Testing & Nutrition: Woodland Publishing, Inc:

161 Murray, M, ND. :Vitamin E: Encyclopedia of Nutritional Supplements: Prima Publishing, P.O. Box 11260BK, Rocklin, CA 9567: PP 49

162 Murray, M, ND. :Diabetes; Encyclopedia of Nutritional Supplements: Prima Publishing, P.O. Box 11260BK, Rocklin, CA 9567: PP 51

163 C-N Lai, Dr.with the Department of Biology, The University of Texas System Cancer Center, part of the M.D. Anderson Hospital & Tumor Institute in Houston, reported in *Nutrition & Cancer* (1:27-30, 1978)

164 Lambert V, Chlorella: the superfood that helps fight disease: Telegraph. Co.UK; Telegraph Media Group Limit, United Kingdom, Published August 17, 2009

165 Howell, E. MD, : Introduction: Unlocking the Secrets of Eating Right For Health, Vitality and Longevity Enzyme Nutrition The Food Enzyme Concept; PP 10

166 Howell, E. MD, : Introduction: Unlocking the Secrets of Eating Right For Health, Vitality and Longevity Enzyme Nutrition The Food Enzyme Concept; PP 9

167 Howell, E. MD, : Introduction: Unlocking the Secrets of Eating Right For Health, Vitality and Longevity Enzyme Nutrition The Food Enzyme Concept; PP 10

168 Bensky, D; Barolet, R: Six-Ingredient Pill with Rehmannia (Liu Wei Di Huang Wan); Eastland Press, Inc, P.O. Box 12689, Seattle, Washington, 98111: PP 263

169 Bensky, D; Barolet, R: Restore the Right (Kidney) Pill (You Gui Wan); Eastland Press, Inc, P.O. Box 12689, Seattle, Washington, 98111: PP 278

170 Bensky, D; Barolet, R: Return the Spleen Decoction (Gui Pi Tang), Eastland Press, Inc, P.O. Box 12689, Seattle, Washington, 98111: PP 255

171 Blach, P., CNC: Fenugreek; Prescription for Herbal Healing; Penguin Putnam, Inc 375 Hudson Street, New York, NY 10014: PP

172

173 Kliment, D.F.:Fats and Oils for the Grain Eater:The Acid Alkaline Balance Diet an innovative Program for Ridding Your Body of Acisic Wastes: Mcgraw-Hill, two Penn Plaza, New York, NY, 10121-2298

174 Website: American Diabetes Association

175 Carper, J: Apple; The Food Pharmacy Dramatic New Evidence That Food Is Your Best Medicine: Bantam Books, 666 Fifth Avenue, New York, NY 10103: PP116

176 Yeager, S: Beans; The Doctors Book of Food Remedies: Rodale Inc: PP 65

177 Blach, P,. CNC, Blach, J., M.D. Spirulina; Prescription for Nutritional Healing; Third Edition: Penguin Putnam Inc.375 Hudson Street, New York, NY 10014: PP 80

178 Ayehunie, S, *etal* " Inhibition of HIV-1 Replication by an Aqueous Extract of Spirulina Platensis (Arthrospira platensis)." JIAD: Journal of Acquired Immune Deficiency Syndromes & Human Retrovirology, 12,1, May 1998: 7-12

179 IIMSAM: www.iimsam.org

180 Whitaker, J. M.D., exercise: A Powerful Therapy for Diabetes; Reversing Diabetes Reduce or Even Eliminate Your Dependence on Insulin or Oral Drugs: Time Warner Book Group, 1271 Avenue of the Americas, New York, NY 10020

181 Johnson, J, A, PhD, DTCM, DMQ(China):Introduction to Medical Qigong Chinese Medical Qigong Therapy A Comprehensive Clinical Text: The International Institute of Medical Qigong, P.O. Box 52144, Pacific grove, CA 93950 USA:PP 5

182 Johnson, J, A, PhD, DTCM, DMQ(China): Introduction to Medical Qigong Chinese Medical Qigong Therapy A Comprehensive Clinical Text: The International Institute of Medical Qigong, P.O. Box 52144, Pacific Grove, CA 93950 USA:PP 14

183 The Value of Qigong in the Management of Diabetes: The C.A.M Report Website: www.thecamreport.com.

184 Flaws, B. Sionneau, P: Diabetes Mellitus: The Treatment of Mordern Western Medical Diseases with Chinese Medicine; A Textbook and Clinical Manual: Blue Poppy Press; a Division of Blue Poppy Enterprise, Inc 5441 Western Ave, Suite 2, Boulder, Co 80301:209

185 Hammer, I.L: The Traditional Five Phase System: Emotion and The Disease Process: Dragon Rise, Red Brid Flies Psychology & Chinese Medicine; revised edition: Eastland Press, Incorporated, P.O. Box 99749, Seattle, Wa 98139 USA: PP 59

186 Hammer, I.L: The Traditional Five Phase System: Emotion and The Disease Process: Dragon Rise, Red Brid Flies Psychology & Chinese Medicine; revised edition: Eastland Press, Incorporated, P.O. Box 99749, Seattle, Wa 98139 USA: PP 62

187 Flaw, B, Kuchinski, L, Casanas, R, M.D.: The Disease Causes & Mechanisms of Diabetes: A textbook and Clinical Manual: Blue Poppy Press A Division of Blue Poppy Enterprises, Inc, 5441 Western Ave, Suite 2, Boulder, CO 80301: PP 22

188 Flaws, B, Sionneau, P: Diabetes Mellitus: The Treatment of Modern Western Medical Diseases with Chinese Medicine: Blue Poppy Press A Division of Blue Poppy Enterprises, Inc, 5441 Western Ave, Suite 2, Boulder, CO 80301: PP 11

189 Flaws, B, Sionneau, P: Diabetes Mellitus: The Treatment of Modern Western Medical Diseases with Chinese Medicine: Blue Poppy Press A Division of Blue Poppy Enterprises, Inc, 5441 Western Ave, Suite 2, Boulder, CO 80301: PP 211

190 Maciocia, G., The Function of the Internal Organs: The Foundations of Chinese Medicine; a Comprehensive Text for Acupuncturists and Herbalists; Second Edition: Elsevier's Health sciences Rights Department, Philadelphia, PA, USA

191 Hammer, L,. M.D., Pychosomatic Medicine: West and East; Dragon Rise, Red Bird Flies:Eastland Press, Incororated, P.O. Box 99749, Seattle, WA 98139 USA : PP54

192 Hammer, L,. M.D., Pychosomatic Medicine: West and East; Dragon Rise, Red Bird Flies:Eastland Press, Incororated, P.O. Box 99749, Seattle, WA 98139 USA : PP73

193 Maciocia, G. CAc,; The Functions of the Large Intestine; The Foundations of Chinese Medicine A Comprehensive Text for Acupuncturists and Herbalist; PP196

194 Maciocia G. The Function of the Kidneys; Foundations of Chinese Medicine A Comprehensive Text for Acupuncture and Herbalists: Elsevier's Health Sciences; Philadelphia, PA, USA: PP513

195 Maciocia G. The Function of the Kidneys; Foundations of Chinese Medicine A Comprehensive Text for Acupuncture and Herbalists: Elsevier's Health Sciences; Philadelphia, PA, USA:PP 154

196 Flaws,B., Kuchinski,L,. Casanas, R. MD, Gestational Diabetes; The Treatment of Diabetes Mellitus with Chinese Medicine; Blue Poppy Press5441 Western Ave, Suite 2 Boulder, CO 80301

197 Hammer, L,. MD., Anxiety and Depression; Dragon Rises, Red Bird Flies Psychology & Chinese Medicine: Eastland Press Incorporated, P. O. Box 99749, Seattle, Wa98139 USA: PP 269

198 Hammer, L,. MD., Water: Mother of the Wood Element; Dragon Rises, Red Bird Flies Psychology & Chinese Medicine: Eastland Press Incorporated, P. O. Box 99749, Seattle, Wa98139 USA: PP 71

199 Whitaker, J. M.D., exercise: A Powerful Therapy for Diabetes; Reversing Diabetes Reduce or Even Eliminate Your Dependence on Insulin or Oral Drugs: Time Warner Book Group, 1271 Avenue of the Americas, New York, NY 10020

Formulas and protocols can be purchased from Healenarts, LLC. Dr. Akmal Muwwakkil is available for book signings, lectures, workshops and trainings.
301-249-2445 Email: akmalmuwwakkil@yahoo.com
Website: healen.net or healenarts.net

Edwards Brothers,Inc!
Thorofare, NJ 08086
04 March, 2011
BA2011063